How to increase your energy, cure poor health and enjoy living longer!

An informative and practical guide on achieving radiant health and longevity through the consumption of certain vital nutrients. <u>These nutrients renew and heal the body as if by magic!</u>

TROY SAWYER

*Special and sincere thanks to Dr Sasha Wasley
and my beautiful wife Lisa for the proof-reading
and editing of this book.*

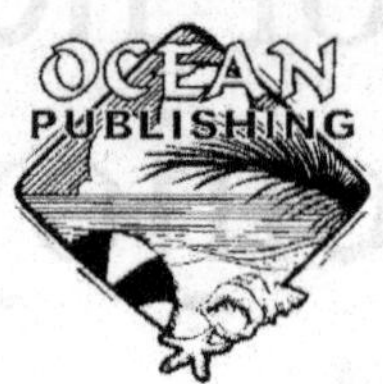

ISBN 978-0-6486196-0-4

Newly revised and updated second edition.

Typesetting and cover design by Steve Barwick.

Full Disclaimer

All information in this book is provided as a general guide only. The author does not imply or express anything regarding the accuracy or reliability of this information or its suitability for a particular purpose.

The author has made every effort to ensure the information contained in this book is correct and they expressly disclaim any reliability or responsibility for the accuracy in this book or for any loss, inconvenience or injury by any person using this book. It is your responsibility to confirm the currency, validity and suitability of all information offered herein.

The author does not make any express or implied warranties, representations or endorsements whatsoever (including, without limitation, the implied warranties of merchantability or fitness for a particular purpose) with regard to the book, the materials, any products, information or service provided throughout the book, or any services listed therein, and the author will not be liable for any cost or damage arising either directly or indirectly from the use of this book.

Meet The Author

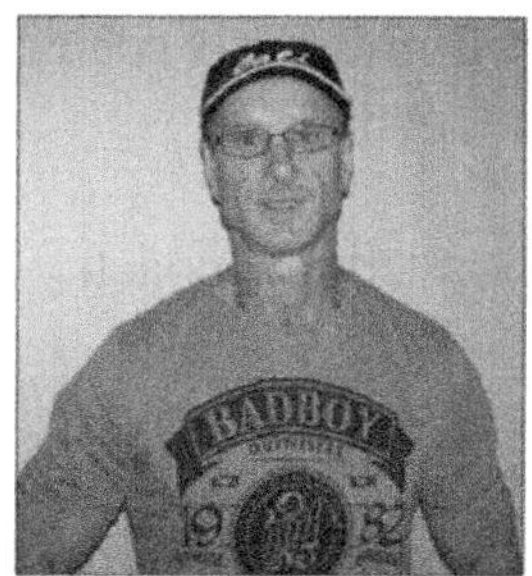

After being struck down with a severe and debilitating illness at the age of 25 and told by medical doctors that little more could be done for him, Troy Sawyer decided to find his own cure through natural recovery methods.

Following several years of extensive research and study into nutritional therapies, he discovered that a deficiency of certain essential nutrients was the cause of his illness. He also discovered that over 90% of diseases are caused by a lack of these essential nutrients and that science has now been able to *prove* that health and longevity is virtually impossible if the body doesn't receive these nutrients on a daily basis.

The problem, however, is as a result of the radical changes in farming methods used today, the food we eat no longer supplies us with enough of these important nutrients. In Troy's case, he had always eaten healthy, yet still became sick. Only after he began to include certain nutritional supplements and vita-nutrients in his diet did he regain his health.

Today, at 55 years young, Troy enjoys the kind of vibrant health and sense of well-being that most people long for and has dedicated the last 25 years to helping others achieve the same.

Some of Troy's qualifications include:

- Certified holistic nutritionist specialising in herbs and nutritional supplements;

- Certified health and wellness coach;

- Certified sports nutritionist;

- Certified personal trainer; and

- Fully qualified lifeguard.

Troy also continues to further his knowledge and stay up-to-date with all of the latest happenings and trends in the natural health field by regularly attending various courses and online workshops. His popular website... **www.lifesavinghealth.org** ranks in the top 1% of all active websites on the internet and provides a wealth of information on various natural remedies and alternative health modalities.

Dedication

This book is dedicated to some very special people in my life. Some who are still living physically and some who have moved on.

Firstly, to the love of my life and my best friend, Lisa. Your patience and sacrifice during the writing and researching of this book was amazing. Never once did you complain. You did, however, provide plenty of encouragement when I needed it. I love you with all my heart.

To my kids, Dianne, Daniel and Amy. Thank you for being the wonderful young people you are and helping to teach me what I need to learn about parenting, in all aspects, good and bad. I love you guys.

To my beautiful grand kids, Natasha, Hayley and Dominic. Your presence always brightens my day and puts a smile on my face. Spending time with you guys makes me realize what's really important in life.

To my Mum and Dad. Thank you so much for instilling in me, and showing through your own actions, that you don't accomplish anything in life without hard work. I love you both.

To my close friend, Gavin Capes. Your passing changed me forever and taught me so much about life and finding my purpose. You dedicated yourself to "protect and serve" humanity. I hope I am able to do that also, in a different way, through this book. I miss you, my friend.

Finally, to my one and only "Poppa" Jack Hicks. The most stubborn and proud man I ever knew. Thank you for passing those traits on down to me or I probably would have never finished this book! You will always stay close to my heart and live in my memories forever.

Troy Sawyer
November 15, 2023

Acknowledgements

I would like to acknowledge and thank one of the true modern pioneers of nutritional therapy, Dr Joel Wallach. The difference you are making to people's health and quality of life is certainly "a breath of fresh air" and long overdue.

Thank you to Les and Patti Dyne for your magnificent contribution to the health and well-being of humanity and the environment.

I would also like to acknowledge and deeply thank some of the other people (past and present) who have been out there helping to spread the word about nutritional therapies, alternative medicines and the bias and corruption that's going on within the pharmaceutical and medical fields. These people include: Ty and Charlene Bollinger, Dr Rashid Buttar, Dr Robert Scott Bell, Robert Kennedy Jr, Dr Carolyn Dean, Dr Garry Gordon, Leigh Erin Connealy M.D., Dr Joseph Mercola, Dr Mark Hyman, Robert Pell, Rick Simpson, Erin Elizabeth, Dr Mary Ruth Swope, David Darbro M.D., Vaughan Bullivant N.D., Dr Gerhard Schrauzer, Robert Barefoot, Dr Bert L'Abbe, Dr Chuck Connery, Dr Yoshihide Hagiwara, Raymond Strand M.D., Ronald Seibold M.S., Webster Kehr, Dr Howard Posner, Bill Anton B. Sc, Dr Gabriel Cousens, Carlos Garcia M.D., Dr Bruce Fife, Dr Patrick Quillin, and Dr Robert Bender.

Many of these people have been severely ridiculed, threatened with having their medical licences revoked and being sued for actively speaking out, yet they continue to show enormous courage by working to expose the truth.

So, to each and every one of you wonderful people, I salute you!

Table of Contents

Introduction

So, why write a book on "how to increase your energy, cure poor health and enjoy living longer"?

Well, if you talk to people, you'll find that these three things are what *every* person wants!

I have not met anyone who has said they could not do with having increased energy, being free from illness and poor health, and enjoying longevity.

In fact, the number one complaint doctors hear from their patients is that they're suffering from a lack of energy. And the number one reason why people visit a doctor in the first place is because of an illness and/or poor health problem.

Recent health studies have also shown that people want to live longer, healthier lives.

Health Myths Exposed...

I think most people today are becoming aware that they are in far less than good health. Health and fitness clubs have become extremely popular as people by the truckloads try to lose weight and get into shape. The nutritional supplement market and the health food market have now developed into booming billion-dollar industries.

We are also being constantly bombarded with advertisements on the need to include more healthy foods such as fresh fruit and vegetables in our diet, and to exclude or cut down on the unhealthy ones like junk food and fatty foods. Many food companies are now even adding vitamins and minerals to certain processed foods such as breakfast cereals, milk and bread.

So why is it that even in spite of all this, people are still complaining about low energy levels and experiencing poor health? And why is it that we are not living even close to our genetic potential?

Well, those questions, along with the plethora of "health myths" that are out there, are precisely what this book will endeavour to explain and answer.

A Taste of What to Expect...

Through this book you will learn 5 little-known (and little practised) health principles. Follow these principles and perfect health is virtually assured.

Here's what else you'll discover:

how you can achieve the ultimate in health and longevity using natural foods (the way that nature intended us to);

how you can sustain maximum energy levels throughout the day without relying on stimulants;

why disease and sickness have become so rampant in society today, and more importantly, how you can prevent and even cure these afflictions;

which specific nutrients you require everyday for health and longevity and how you can obtain them easily and inexpensively;

how you can finally put an end to the diet merry go round and reach and maintain your ideal body weight for good;

the natural antibiotic and virtual "cure all" you can take that's

10 times more powerful (and safer) than any pharmaceutical drug; and

how your brain and what you feed it plays a crucial role in your overall health (and can even determine your lifespan).

The list certainly goes on... but suffice it to say that by the time you've finished reading this book, you'll have the knowledge and information you need to go on and enjoy living the long and healthful life you've always wanted to live... with plenty of vitality and energy to match!

Reliable Information...

The information you'll find presented in this book is fully referenced and has come from a variety of dependable and sound sources.

Most of this information is supported by scientific studies and research that has been performed and documented over the past 90 years. Much of it is the direct result of the ground-breaking and dedicated work of some of the finest people who have ever been involved in the fields of nutrition, health, and longevity.

I do not claim any credit for the information contained in this book. The credit must go to the people and the research institutions who, through their amazing work over almost a century, have helped to make this information become - and continue to become – widely accepted right around the world.

You may also notice that many of the studies referenced in this book are "older" studies. There is a reason for this. Unfortunately, the majority of studies performed today are funded by pharmaceutical companies or powerful entities that have a vested interest in poo-pooing or discrediting any natural alternative that may get in the way of their pharmaceutical product.

Bogus and rigged studies are rife today. This is sad but true.

The "older" verified studies were not subject to this deception and are much more reliable in my view, hence why I reference many of these. Remember, a study result from 20 years ago is the same as what it is today. The outcome and benefit do not change!

An Easy Read Reference Guide...

You will find this book written in a very simple, easy-to-read style and a me-to-you type manner. To me, there's nothing worse (or more boring) than trying to read an information-based book and finding you need to be a scientist or a college professor to understand it all.

So I have tried, where possible, to avoid a lot of the scientific jargon and complicated information that can sometimes be associated with the subject of health and nutrition by sticking with the "KISS" principal (keep it simple, stupid).

I like the idea that if a twelve-year-old can't understand it then neither will an adult!

Expert Opinions will Differ

I am well aware that there's going to be some (or all) of the information contained in this book that many of the "experts" will not agree with. So be it.

Because nutrition and nutritional therapy is such a vast and somewhat complex subject (and at times conflicting), there are a lot of differences-of-opinion within the health and medical industries. Not everyone agrees on the same points (mind you, you get that with anything in life, don't you?) Unfortunately, many of these "experts" seem to believe they have all the answers and their way is the only way.

What I have hopefully been able to do with this book is present the information that I have gathered and give it to you in a simple, honest and relatively unbiased way. After you read it, you can then make up your own mind as to whether you think it will be of benefit to you.

I certainly do not claim to have all the answers, nor do I think my way is the only way. I do wholeheartedly believe, however, that my way is one darn good way that gets results!

Time is of the Essence...

Well, I'm not only "jumping out of my skin" with excitement at being able to share this important and what I feel is lifesaving information with you, I also feel a tremendous sense of urgency in doing so.

You see, I think it's time we all faced up to one simple truth, and that is this... the health and well-being of the human race is really suffering badly today, no doubt about it. We have somehow gone and forgotten the natural laws and ways of nature and, unfortunately, are now paying for it dearly.

I am confident, however, that we can all turn our health and well-being around simply by following some basic principles, which will be revealed to you throughout this book.

So please read on and find out how you can increase your energy, cure poor health and enjoy living longer. I guarantee that once you do, you'll never want to go back to your old tired, unhealthy self again!

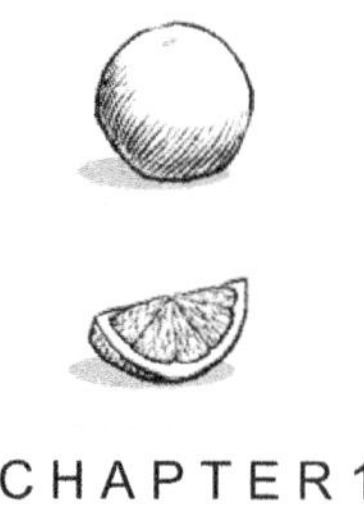

A Brief Story: From Debilitating Illness to Renewed Health...

What would you say is the greatest asset you can have in life?

Actually, before you go and answer that question, let's first define the word "asset," which literally means "something of value."

Now, I know the answer might be different for a lot of people, but most would probably say material possessions such as owning your own home, money or financial security. At least these are what we are constantly being told are the most important assets to have. And I would certainly agree that in today's world these are important, but they are still so far second to the one thing that most people seem to always overlook... *your health!*

Think about this: everyone you talk to dreams of winning the lottery, don't they? If only their numbers would come up then all of their troubles would be over – or so they think.

Well, what if you did happen to win and you were able to enjoy all the wealth and prosperity you wanted, but you didn't have your health to go with it?

Would it be worth it? — I don't think so.

You wouldn't be fit enough, or around long enough to enjoy it all anyway!

As the great Izaak Walton once said: *"Health is ... a blessing that money cannot buy."* [2]

I always remember reading an article about legendary singer Sir Paul McCartney and how shattered he was when his first wife, Linda – whom he says was the love of his life – died of breast cancer.

Now, here's a man who at the time, seemingly had everything in life he could ever want and wish for. Everything except the woman he loved and adored that is.

All of that wealth and prosperity still couldn't save his wife.

Paul was at Linda's bedside when she passed and I bet at that moment, and even for a long while after, he would have gladly given up every asset, everything he had and possessed in an instant to have her back again.

Make no mistake, your health and your family's health are the most valuable assets and prized possessions you could ever have – bar none!

You Don't Know What You've got Until it's Gone

What I find really amazing is how people will have their lists of priorities and goals to achieve in life all set out, and yet their health and taking care of their bodies (which is the vehicle that's going to carry them there) is totally neglected and taken for granted. In fact, most people take better care of their garden or their pets than they do their own health!

The other sad fact is a lot of people *think* they're taking care of their health by eating foods they have been told to eat by doctors, nutritionists and other so-called experts, yet they continue to feel lethargic and experience poor health (two definite signs that something is wrong). This is what happened to me back in 1993 at the tender age of 25…

I was what some people might describe as an over-the-top health nut and gym junkie. At this point in time, I was in serious training, working out at the gym five to six times a week (something I had been doing for the past eight years) and eating what I thought was a perfectly planned and healthy diet (i.e., eating from the four/five basic food groups like we've been told to do, no junk food, no refined foods, no alcohol, and so on).

I was so health conscious that I wouldn't even take an aspirin if I had a headache. I would just put up with the pain!

However, in spite of this so-called "healthy lifestyle," I was suddenly struck down with Chronic Fatigue Syndrome (CFS). I didn't even know what CFS was at that stage. It was still a relatively new type of ailment back then. All I remembered was what I'd heard from a well-known champion cyclist, who had been suffering from the disease, when he was talking about it on the television a few months earlier.

CFS is Nasty!

Unfortunately, because of our poor eating habits and the lack of nutrients contained in our foods today, Chronic Fatigue Syndrome has become a very common illness.

For those of you who you don't know anything about CFS and what it does, it basically makes you feel extremely tired and lethargic and you become very susceptible to other types of illnesses.

In my own case I became extremely fatigued, not only physically, but mentally as well. I couldn't remember things, no matter how hard I tried, and my mind was always "cloudy" and unfocused.

Trying to exercise five times a week became a real struggle. In fact, just trying to get through the day was a huge struggle!

On top of this, I had two serious bouts of Glandular Fever within six-months of each other and it seemed as though whenever a cold or flu virus was going around, I was always the first one to get it. I got to a point where I was sick and tired of being sick and tired! (I know many people can relate to this).

The Downhill Slide Continued...

In addition to this, I had been suffering for quite some time with a painful and troublesome knee that would just "lock up" if I kept it in the same position for too long. Bending my leg would also produce a very loud grinding and clicking noise and soreness in the joint was always constant, especially during the colder winter months.

After having numerous tests, ultrasounds, x-rays, and even a major operation, doctors told me I had the beginnings of degenerative arthritis and there was nothing I could do to stop it.

I remember wondering at this time that if this was how my knee was at the age of 25, what would it be like by the time I reached age 50? (I would probably need a knee replacement). Mind you, the way my body was continually breaking down back then, I doubt that I would have even made it to fifty!

My declining state of health continued on like this for the next three years. During this time, I tried all sorts of therapies including taking high doses of synthetic vitamins, drinking Kombucha tea, and even sleeping for ten hours a day. All with little success.

I must admit at this stage I did begin to get quite discouraged that nothing was working, but I was determined to keep on searching for a cure.

Giving up just wasn't an option... it couldn't be an option!!

Then, out of the blue, I met someone who began to put me on the right road to recovery.

After inquiring very curiously as to why I was drinking that foul smelling Kombucha tea (if you've ever had it brewing in your house you'll understand) - and me reluctantly telling him why - he handed me a cassette tape (remember those?) and suggested that I'd benefit from listening to it.

On the tape, this Naturopathic doctor was talking about longevity and how to improve your health. It was filled with some amazing information that I'd never heard before and after listening to it the lights in my head went on and the bells started ringing!

From this beginning, I decided to find and study everything I possibly could on natural health and healing. It all became **very** interesting. The right books and the right information began to come into my life exactly as I needed them.

I must point out here that back in 1996 there was no internet, so the only real way that you could research something was by going to your local library and hiring books and tape sets - then reading and listening and taking notes. This was a very slow and tedious process.

Fortunately, you don't have to do this today. Now you have Dr Google!

The Change in my Health was Astonishing

So, what I learnt from Nobel Prize Nominee and renowned

Naturopathic physician, Dr Joel Wallach, was that the human body needs 90 nutrients *every day*, in the right proportions, to function at its peak. [1]

But here's the really interesting part. By making sure you take in these 90 nutrients every day, you can virtually **guarantee** yourself a long and healthy life free of sickness and disease.

I thought straight away... that's definitely for me!

I knew this was what I had to do to get myself healthy, and so I began making sure I received all of these nutrients every day from natural sources such as wheat grass (barley grass), colloidal minerals, a lactobacillus food and evening primrose oil (all of which I'll be explaining about in the coming chapters).

After just 12 weeks I knew I was onto something big. My energy levels were the best they'd been in over five years. People also started to comment on my brighter eyes and how much more alive I looked. I even had some of the ladies I knew, who worked for a major skin care and cosmetic company, asking me what I was using on my skin to keep it looking so good.

Seriously!

I also haven't been sick once in the past 20 years, which is definitely some kind of record for me, and my knee has never felt better. It doesn't lock up any more and the soreness in the joint is completely gone.

My Blood Test was the Real Proof in the Pudding

I really do feel fantastic today, and it's so good to be able to go to the gym and to go for my daily walks and bike rides. I actually enjoy and look forward to exercising now that I have more energy, whereas before I found I just couldn't be bothered.

I also decided to go and have a live blood microscopy done so that I could see exactly what sort of condition my blood, and therefore my body, was in.

These tests can tell you just about everything from the condition of your liver and kidneys, to the number of parasites in the blood, and the healthiness of the red blood cells, white blood cells and plasma.

They're especially effective because the blood is still fresh and alive when it's analyzed, not dead like the common blood tests that are taken by your local M.D. and sent off to a laboratory.

My results? The Naturopath who did the test for me said that out of all the people he had done the live blood microscopy for, <u>my blood was by far the cleanest he had ever seen!</u>

I just wished I had of gone and had the test done *before* I started having my daily supplements. Then I could have seen just how bad it was back then, compared to what it is now.

It Worked for Friends and Family too...

After the positive results I gained from taking the wheat grass, colloidal minerals, lactobacillus food and evening primrose oil, my family and some friends of ours started doing the same thing, with equal results.

Our children had always been labelled as "sickly kids" by doctors and every winter they were always off to our local M.D. for some type of treatment for a viral or bacterial infection. Amazingly, they never had to go back to the doctor for *any* illness in over seven years of taking these supplements, and that includes two winters which saw unprecedented flu and virus epidemics in our community.

Now, I will say that during this time they had once or twice experienced minor ailments such as a runny nose or slight cough, but I was surprised at how quickly these would clear up. Something that normally would last for weeks was gone within a few days.

One of our children was also diagnosed with Attention Deficit Hyperactive Disorder (ADHD) when she was younger.

She was put on the drug Ritalin (we didn't know any better at the time) and although her behaviour and schoolwork did improve, we were not comfortable with our eight-year-old child having to take such a powerful drug every day.

After she'd been having the natural supplements for about four months, we decided to cut out the Ritalin. We began to limit the amount of sugar in her diet as well (which is very important for people with ADHD) and she started taking the herb Gingko Biloba (this herb is renowned for helping people with ADHD as it increases blood flow to the brain).

It worked like a charm. She never had to use the Ritalin from that point on, and incredibly, 18 months later her behaviour and schoolwork were still at the same level of improvement as when she was taking the drug!

Yes, but...

The results were really quite extraordinary and we were ecstatic that she no longer needed the drug.

This all changed however when she decided to go and live with her biological father. She stopped taking the supplements at that time and within the *first* week of starting a new school, her teacher noticed she had an attention problem. Her father took her to see a paediatrician and guess what? He put her back on Ritalin!

In addition to this, her asthma (which had actually stopped during this time) soon returned and she started using a puffer again. She also contracted a serious virus that caused her to have two weeks off school. (To me, this is good evidence of how valuable these nutrients are and just how badly they're lacking from our diets today).

Even More Proof...

I continued to do as much research, and find out as much information as I possibly could, about the nutrients and natural foods we were consuming. The more I researched, the more people I read about who had experienced similar results to our own.

Remarkably, many people had overcome serious illnesses and life-threatening diseases such as cancer by using these natural foods. Some were even considered "terminal" and yet they were able to recover and go on to live normal and productive lives.

Many others I read about were just like the majority of today's population - suffering from general poor-health and lethargy.

And yes, they too were able to benefit tremendously from the daily intake of these nutritional supplements.

The all Important 90 Nutrients...

So what are the 90 nutrients our bodies need every day for optimum health and longevity? In no particular order... we need 60 minerals, 16 vitamins, 12 essential amino acids and 2 essential fatty acids. [1]

Making sure your body receives these nutrients every day is absolutely *critical*. In fact, I like to think of it as a matter of ***life and death!***

I'm sure none of us would ever deliberately try to jeopardise our life or the lives of our loved ones in any way.

However, I believe that is what we are unknowingly doing to ourselves by not making sure we take in these nutrients on a daily basis. And don't think for one second that we're able to get them all from our diet. As you'll discover later, it's now virtually impossible!

The good news though is it's not too late to fix things.

When you start having these foods and supplements on a daily basis, your body will begin to cleanse itself of all the unwanted chemicals and deadly toxins that build up every day, along with repairing the damage that's already been done by renewing and regenerating itself.

Even if your body has been subjected to a lot of use and abuse over the years, you can still reverse the process. You just have to give your body the right raw materials it needs every day to do the job.

I like to think of it in the same way as having a plant, such as a rose bush, growing in your garden. If you neglected that rose bush and didn't feed it what it needed (water and fertilizer) it would slowly wither and begin to die. But if you began to feed and nourish it with the right materials, it would regrow and eventually blossom back into a beautiful and healthy plant.

Your body is designed to do the exact same thing!

* * *

So without giving away *too* much information *too* early, just remember that it's never too late for us to turn our health and well-being around, and we can do this by making sure we feed the body the right nutrients (all 90) it needs every day to cleanse, repair and regenerate itself.

In the next chapter, we're going to look more closely at some of the reasons why we as a society have allowed ourselves to become so unhealthy, and why disease and sickness have now reached epidemic proportions.

We will also endeavour to find out the reasons why preventative approaches are either non-existent today or simply don't work, and why drugs have now become the so-called "cures" for our health problems instead of natural alternatives.

Finally, we'll talk about why it's so important that *you* begin today on the road to good health, vitality and longevity.

Let's continue on, shall we? ...

CHAPTER 2

More "Wonder Drugs" and Medical Procedures Today Yet More Sickness and Disease?

So how much importance do *you* personally, place on your health?

Does it come first in your life, above everything else, or is it something that you don't give much thought to?

Do you tell yourself that "one day" you'll start to take better care of your health? Or maybe you think that you *are* taking care of your health?

And what about your children and your loved ones – how important is their health to you?

I know these may seem like trivial or even silly questions, but I believe you have to answer them seriously (and truthfully) or you'll never make the necessary effort to improve your health.

I find that most people will put up with feeling tired, run down and experiencing poor health because that's the way they think it has to be. They don't know there's an alternative.

I also find that a lot of people will continuously abuse their bodies through various destructive means such as eating unhealthy foods, smoking, drinking alcohol excessively, not getting enough rest, being under constant stress, and so on; yet when they end up with a serious ailment or disease because of these choices they wonder why!

Just remember something else… once you die, your life on this planet is over for you… *for good*. You aren't going to get another chance to repeat it or extend it.

Life is not a dress rehearsal – it's the live stage show!

Why go and throw it away foolishly and prematurely?

I suggest we all live life to the fullest and get the maximum number of years possible out of our bodies.

Regret is an Awful Thing…

It's a known fact that when someone develops a terminal illness that's been caused by something they physically did to themselves (self-inflicted), and therefore could have prevented (smoking, unhealthy eating habits, etc), it's common for that person to feel overwhelming regret for their actions. They know that their poor choices have now cost them their life.

I'd like you to consider this scenario for a moment...

I'd like you to imagine that it's *you* lying there on the bed in a hospital with a terminal disease or illness. With the doctors unable to do anything more for you, you're basically just lying there waiting to die.

Suddenly you think those two regretful words to yourself… "if only":

"If only I had of decided to really take care of my health when I still had the chance, I might have been able to live another 10, 20, maybe even 30 years longer. Maybe then I could have travelled and seen some of the places I've always wanted to see, or done some of the things I've always wanted to do but never found the time. Maybe

I might have even been around to walk my daughter down the aisle or see my grandchildren grow up."

So many people get caught up working towards their "retirement" and getting their superannuation or pension payout so they can do the things they've planned most of their lives for.

But what if you die before you get there?

What a waste!

While I'm on the subject of retirement and living in one's latter years, most people think that as you get older you become more susceptible to certain diseases. That's simply not true.

Well known health crusader and life extension specialist, Paul Bragg, once stated: *"It has definitely been proven by some of the greatest scientific minds in the world that there are no special diseases of old age."* [2]

The truth is *we* allow ourselves to become prone to sickness and disease. The body is a self-healing mechanism. It's designed to heal itself and keep itself healthy, but like I said before, only if you give it the right nutrients it needs every day to cleanse, repair and regenerate itself.

Just like a car that doesn't receive a regular oil change and service will wear out prematurely and eventually break down, so will the human body – except the human body can tolerate abuse for a lot longer. But remember this: if you abuse your body, eventually you will pay the price for your actions.

Maybe even the ultimate price?

Your Body is the Most Amazing Creation...

I think most people would agree that of all the creations in the universe, the human body is by far the greatest. What it achieves over a lifetime is nothing short of astounding.

For instance, the human heart, which is only the size of your fist, can easily pump in excess of 8000 litres of blood per day. In an average person's lifetime that would equate to almost 227 million litres of blood!

The human body contains around 160,000 kilometres (100,000 miles) of blood vessels, which is enough to go around the world four times non-stop. [4]

The average body is also made up of around 37 trillion cells, and these cells are constantly being replaced by new cells. Astonishingly, every 7-10 years you actually end up with a totally *new* body. New arms, legs, hands, feet, and even a new face, even though those new parts look identical to the old ones! [3]

The Survival Statistics...

No machine could ever do what the human body does every day to keep itself alive and functioning. Yet so many people treat their bodies like machines, expecting them to perform at their peak and never break down. When it comes to a serious illness or disease, they seem to have the "it will never happen to me" syndrome.

So, what are the actual chances of someone getting (and possibly dying from) a serious ailment or disease?

If we look at diseases like cancer and heart disease, statistics show that these two alone claim *over 50% of all deaths* in the Western world today. [3]

More "Wonder Drugs" and Medical Procedures Today Yet More Sickness and Disease

In the United States, someone suffers a heart attack every 34 seconds and one out of every three people will die from a heart attack, stroke or related disease (or one every 60 seconds). Heart disease has now become the biggest single cause of early death in America, Great Britain, Australia, and most European countries. [5]

Then we have cancer, which is probably the one disease that scares the heck out of everybody because it's so destructive and cruel. Statistics show that one in three people will get cancer during their lives (soon to be one in two!). Cancer has also become the leading cause of death for children under the age of fifteen. [3]

Unfortunately, these two diseases have become so rampant today that I'm sure we all know or have known at least one person who's been affected by them.

What's interesting to note though is 100 years ago these diseases weren't even prevalent amongst society, yet today they stand out as number one killers.

Other diseases and ailments that were not prevalent 100 years ago, yet today are rampant amongst society include: liver disease, diabetes, high cholesterol, high blood pressure, birth defects, asthma, osteoporosis, arthritis and Alzheimer's disease, just to name a few.

Speaking of Alzheimer's disease, a little over a 100 years ago this disease was totally unheard of (the first documented case was in 1907). Today, one out of every two people who reach age seventy will get Alzheimer's disease. [1]

In addition to this, it's very common to hear people today constantly complaining about health problems such as headaches, backaches, allergies, digestive problems, lack of energy, being overweight, etc. It's almost never ending!

Why are we Going in Reverse?

The obvious question you have to ask yourself is why is it that in this current age of apparent, state-of-the-art, high-tech medicine, do we see more sickness and more disease in the world than ever before?

Why, if we're supposed to be becoming healthier, do countries like the U.S., Great Britain and Australia continue to spend billions and even trillions of dollars on medical care every year (the U.S. is about to hit the 4.5 trillion dollar a year mark). [6]

Why is it, with so much progress supposedly being made in medical science - and with the medical profession boldly claiming to have more answers to our health problems than ever before - do we see hospitals overcrowded and new medical centres being built at a faster rate than ever before?

And why is it that a country like America, which focuses on conventional medicine and accounts for over *half* of all money spent in the world on health care, rank a dismal 24th in the world on longevity out of 28 industrialized nations according to a World Health Organization survey? If conventional medicine was the answer to our health crisis, then they should rank at the top, or at least near the top, shouldn't they? [7]

I believe the problem with all of this is we as human beings have for some reason changed our way of thinking over the years. We have moved away from natural treatments and natural remedies. Instead, we now turn to surgery and pharmaceutical drugs to try and cure our diseases and health problems.

But the truth is, drugs rarely cure anything. In fact, according to prominent doctor, Dr Howard Posner... *"They just suppress the causes and symptoms while the underlying problem or disease continues to go on."* [7]

As for surgery – it's very rarely a long term fix. Many patients actually come away from surgery worse off than when they went in.

Some don't even make it out of the hospital!

In a disturbing report by Ralph Naitor and Sydney Wolf, it was discovered that in America alone 150,000 to 300,000 people are *killed* each year in hospitals as a result of medical negligence. Yes, that's right, 150,000 to 300,000. [9]

Be sure to keep that statistic in mind the next time your doctor wants to cut you open and tells you it's a safe or "routine" procedure!

The Problem with Pharmaceuticals...

Today, many doctors seem to be baffled as to the reasons why our health is continuing to decline, and why disease and sickness are now rampant amongst society.

The medical profession still continues to focus on finding so-called "cures" with pharmaceutical drugs which, in many cases, can be even more harmful to our health than the ailment we're suffering from.

Even drugs like aspirin and sleeping pills, which are considered mild, can put extra stress on bodily organs like the liver and kidneys.

Then there's harder drugs like HRT (Hormone Replacement Therapy) which has been found to increase breast cancer in women by 78% and increase cardio vascular disease by a whopping 200% (HRT is still being prescribed, by the way). And what about the awful Vioxx drug that killed 139,000 people in America alone.[10] New findings on the 'love making drug" Viagra have found that it can now cause men to go blind (yes, I know, they say that too much sex will make you go blind anyway!).

Current statistics show that **less than 20%** of the drugs that are administered by physicians today are even effective. But that's okay; at least the almighty drug companies (which are some of the most powerful and influential companies in the world) are still making billions of dollars profit each year. [11]

I don't know about you, but I'm also growing tired of hearing about the latest medical research or medical breakthrough that "shows real promise" (they all seem to show promise yet few actually deliver).

The problem is people get their hopes up for a cure and then find the drug or treatment doesn't live up to its original expectation.

A prime example of this is chemotherapy. When this was first introduced it was being hailed as a state-of-the-art "wonder treatment" for cancer. The reality of it now is much different.

Most people are unaware that the 5 year survival rate of a cancer patient treated with chemotherapy is only a dismal 2.1% in the United States and 2.3% in Australia. So, in other words, 5 years after treatment, 97.9% of cancer patients who listened to their doctor and went with the chemo will not be alive! If you don't believe me, go on the NCBI (PubMed) government website and see the results of the study for yourself. Just search... "Contribution of Cytotoxic Chemotherapy to 5-year Survival in Adult Malignancies". [52]

I also remember reading about the drug Cortisone and when that was first introduced. This one was going to be a certain cure for arthritis.

Not so of course.

Although it can block out the pain caused from arthritis, the devastating side effects (such as severely suppressing the immune system, pulling minerals from the bones, increasing the rate of diabetes, and wearing the joints away faster[9]) far outweigh any potential benefits in my view.

Then there's the latest weight loss drugs that have hit the market.

There was so much hype over these and everyone thought they were going to be the ultimate diet pills, yet not one has lived up to its original expectation.

Now don't get me wrong, I do believe that certain drugs have their place in medicine and can be worthwhile and beneficial. The problem though is pharmaceuticals are simply used *way* too much today, and in many cases, are dished out to patients like lollies.

It's also amazing just how many people will visit their doctor for a minor ailment and be given a very powerful drug to treat that ailment.

Prevention is the Key...

I guess you're probably starting to realise that I'm not a big fan of conventional medicine.

I am, however, a strong advocate for natural cures and natural treatments, which I believe are a far better alternative to conventional medicine, and don't come with harmful side effects.

But even better than all of these is *prevention*. Giving your body what it needs every day so you won't need any cures or treatments!

Here's an interesting quote I found whilst writing this book: *"Our medical technology is by far the most advanced, but our preventative approaches are by far the worst."* [3]

How true that is?

I remember my grandmother at age 60 telling me she asked her doctor whether it was worth her taking nutritional supplements to help prevent any illness or disease?

He told her flatly, "They're a waste of time!"

What really concerned me about this is not only did this doctor obviously know very little about prevention, but he's also someone in the community that people look up to and naturally expect that he has the answers to their health problems. Most people would take his advice without questioning it because he's a "doctor."

Fortunately, my grandmother didn't listen to him and she lived to be a healthy 91 years of age!

We Still Need Doctors

Now I know it's beginning to sound like I'm dead against doctors and what they do – but I'm not. I really think most of them do a wonderful job and should be commended for the work they do and the many lives they save, especially when it comes to an emergency or life-threatening situation.

Without them we would definitely be worse off that's for sure.

At the same time, I think G.P.'s and M.D.'s need to be very careful about the advice they give to their patients. They don't receive any formal training in nutrition and nutritional therapies so I don't believe they should give people advice on the subject.

It's actually interesting to note, by the way, that doctors only live to an average age of fifty-six, whereas the rest of the population live to an average age of seventy five (strange how we listen to and take advice from people who live on average fewer years than we do?). [1]

I would certainly welcome the day that doctors had to receive formal training in nutritional therapies as well as orthodox (conventional) medicine.

In fact, one of the worlds true "geniuses" Thomas Edison once said:

> *The doctor of the future will give no medicine, but will interest his patients in the care of the human frame, in diet, and in the cause and prevention of disease.* [2]

Thankfully, there **are** doctors today who are moving away from orthodox medical treatments and are now focusing more on natural alternatives, although they are not welcomed by the medical profession. Many of these doctors are seen as "quacks" and "traitors" by fellow medical practitioners and the A.M.A (American Medical Association), who seem to believe that conventional medicine is the be all and end all to our health problems.

As one certified "quack", Dr David Darbro, explains:

Much of what I've learned since my "awakening" has to do with using nutrition as medicine. This is what makes the average M.D. hot under the collar. He isn't opposed to good nutrition, it's just that he doesn't see it having anything to do with the practice of medicine. The idea of helping the body in a general way rather than combating a specific problem in the body is totally foreign to him. Furthermore, his training taught him that "scientific proof" is necessary to validate everything. If it's not in his medical literature, it's not any good. So clinical nutrition, herbal remedies, drugless medicine, and the like, are worthless to him because there's no "proof" they work – no proof that is, in his sense of the word. He cares nothing for the fact that the patients get better – getting better isn't scientific enough. It defies his logic. [12]

It's wonderful to see that Naturopaths and other alternative health practitioners are becoming increasingly popular today and many people are even consulting them for their health problems *first* – rather than doctors.

There's a popular trend developing towards alternative medicine. I think that people are becoming very disillusioned with conventional medicine and are beginning to wonder whether this type of treatment is the answer to their health problems.

They are also becoming aware that drugs can be harmful and have side effects, some of them serious.

Natural medicine, on the other hand, is safe; and because more and more people are experiencing positive results from this, its popularity is growing rapidly!

Our Health Crisis Revealed...

Going back to what I spoke about earlier, there really is no great mystery as to why the health of the nation - and the world for that matter - is declining so rapidly and why disease and sickness have continued to escalate over the years. Many health experts have now come to the conclusion that: *"Our increasingly deficient food supplies are the true cause of much of our suffering."* [13]

Studies have consistently shown that the nutritional quality of the fruits, vegetables and grains we're eating have steadily declined over the past 150 years. Today we are eating nothing but "nutrient dead" foods. [47]

What's more, according to Dr Joel Wallach, it's been proven through autopsy studies that people who die of so-called "natural causes" actually die of a *nutritional deficiency!* [9]

Remember that our bodies need 90 nutrients every day for optimal health and longevity. Because this is not happening, illness and disease are flourishing, people are experiencing low energy levels - and of course, we are not living even close to our genetic potential.

So why has the nutritional quality of the foods we're eating declined so much over the years?

There are several reasons.

The first, and probably the biggest, are the farming methods and the way in which these have changed over the past 150 years. The crops (and yields) that farmers used to produce 150 years ago were "mineral rich" bumper crops.

What exactly do I mean by this?

Well, first you need to understand that plants (which of course includes fruits, vegetables and grains) cannot make minerals in the same way they can manufacture vitamins, amino acids and fatty acids. Minerals have to _first_ be in the soil, then the plant is able to absorb them up through their root system and store them (in organic form) for their own use. We then come along and eat these mineral rich plants and gain the health benefits.

This is what was happening back 150 years ago.

Unfortunately, though, no minerals were being put back into the soil, and because down through the generations farmers began to graze on the same land year after year, these crops slowly became "mineral deficient" (it only takes 5-10 years to completely leach all minerals from the soil).[1]

Sadly, our food crops today are virtually stripped of all essential minerals.

You see, the problem is farmers don't get paid to put minerals back in the soil, they only get paid for tonnes and bushels per acre of crop. All that interests them is being able to produce a bumper crop with a minimum amount of cost.

So, what they use is a commercial fertilizer called NPK or super phosphate. This fertilizer is very cost efficient for farmers and is the only nutrition plants actually need to grow and appear healthy (notice I use the word "appear").

The major problem for us health wise is this fertilizer only contains two minerals and one element (nitrogen, phosphorous and potassium). The other 58 minerals we need aren't there!

An article in the *Journal of Ecology of Disease* stated: *"Without a doubt the health of both animals and men is linked to the mineral balance of their soils."* And back in 1993, the *World Health Organization* actually came out and said that 95% of our soils are now depleted (makes you wonder how much worse they are today?). [14]

Essential Vitamins, Amino Acids and Fatty Acids are Also Missing...

Another major problem is because the soil our produce is grown on is severely deficient in minerals and organic matter (including essential organisms), this also affects the plant being able to manufacture vitamins, amino acids and fatty acids.

As a result, these are now lacking significantly in our foods.

Recent studies that have been carried out on our different foods and published in various magazines and journals, including a great article in *Natural Life Review* magazine titled, *How Nutritious is Your Food,* have confirmed this shocking trend. [15]

Here's something else to think about...

We're told by The Heart Foundation, The Cancer Council and other health institutes to include plenty of fresh fruits and vegetables in our diet to stay healthy and prevent disease. How is this going to be of any real benefit when there's barely any nutrition left in the foods we're buying from the supermarket?

For instance, we're told to eat spinach for iron.

You would need to consume a huge amount of spinach every day to get an adequate supply of your daily iron.

We then go and cook our food which then destroys any vitamins, amino acids, fatty acids and live enzymes that may be in these foods anyway (the only way to make sure your body receives the valuable nutrients it needs every day is to supplement with organic "nutrient rich" foods such as wheat grass and plant based colloidal minerals).

Cancer Causing Pesticides and Chemicals

Another alarming fact is the amount of artificial pesticides that are used on our food crops today. These pesticides then end up in the foods we eat.

It's now been proven that these chemicals alter the genes of the body, which means we then become more susceptible to killer diseases like cancer.

I remember as a child my mother telling me to always wash fruit and vegetables before eating them to remove any chemicals. I now realize this didn't help all that much because the chemicals actually go *inside* these foods as well as outside, the same way that any chemical will go into the body through the pores of the skin if we come into contact with it.

Then, if having our produce doused with chemicals is not enough, food companies go and add even more chemicals and artificial food additives to our processed and manufactured foods (there are about 4000 artificial chemicals and food additives in our food chain today). *We are literally being poisoned every time we eat!* [4]

So how can we try to avoid ingesting these chemicals?

Reading labels on the foods you buy in the supermarket so you know what artificial additives are in them is a good start. Also trying to eat natural foods that are free of additives and organically grown will certainly help as well.

Remember, any way we can help to reduce the amount of chemicals going into our bodies is definitely going to benefit us in the long run.

But Wait, There's More...

I wish I could stop there, but sadly the "chemical drenching" we receive doesn't end with the foods we eat.

Every day we're also subjected to more chemicals and pollutants from the environment, the worst being diesel fumes, which have been found to be one of the most carcinogenic (cancer causing) of all.

Other harmful chemicals are contained in personal care products like shampoos, deodorants, soaps, household products and detergents. As I said, these chemicals are absorbed through the pores of the skin, straight into the bloodstream.

Needless to say, trying to avoid all of these chemicals every day is extremely difficult (virtually impossible really) and remember that once in the body, they do have the potential to cause serious health problems.

But there is good news on the subject because taking live foods such as wheat grass or barley grass will detoxify and flush (chelate) these chemicals out of the body.

So even though it may be difficult to avoid ingesting and coming into contact with these chemicals, at least we can safely remove them every day. This way, they will not accumulate and become harmful and cause cancer and other serious health problems in years to come.

* * *

Alright, now that we know some of the reasons *why* we are experiencing health problems today, and how we can begin to fix them so we can prevent ill health and enjoy living healthier lives, it's almost time to cover the crucial 90 nutrients we need in more detail.

But before we do that, I would like to briefly share with you some interesting information on longevity, which will prove to you once and for all that we can prevent disease and live longer by taking in these nutrients every day.

The sad fact is we are living way short of our genetic potential compared to some cultures in the world, and in the next chapter, we're going to find out the reasons why they enjoy longevity and we don't.

Let's keep going...

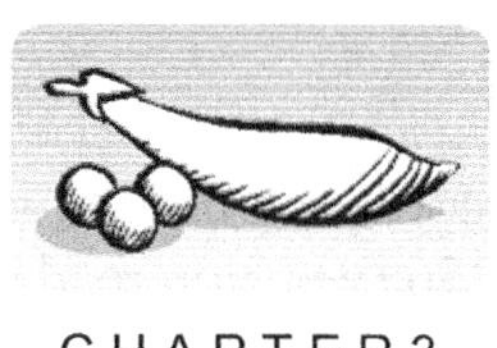

CHAPTER 3

Longevity... Secrets to Living
to a Healthy 100 Years and Beyond...

When someone in the Western world reaches 100 years of age, we think of that as a super human effort, don't we?

We would even consider them to be extremely "lucky" – after all, not many people get to reach the magic three figures.

But the human body is genetically designed to last for a lot longer than 100 years.

Do you know how many years it might be?

This may surprise you, but scientists have been able to prove that the genetic potential for longevity for a human being is between 120 and 140 years (minimum). [9]

That's how long our bodies are actually meant to last for!

Yet in the Western World the average lifespan for a human is around 75 years, only about half of our genetic potential.

I find this information fascinating because there's at least five cultures in the world where their people routinely live to be 120 to 140 years of age – so it's not just a theory, it's a very real possibility. [9,13]

The most famous of these would have to be the Russian Georgians and the Tibetans in Western China. As a matter of fact, Dr Li Chung

47

Yun, who lived along the Tibetan border, is believed to have lived until the ripe old age of 256 (yes, you read correctly!). [3]

Other cultures that also enjoy longevity include the Hunzas in Eastern Pakistan, the Armenians in the former Soviet Union, the Titicacans in Peru and the Azerbaijanis in the Middle East.

Speaking of the Azerbaijanis, in January of 1973 an article appeared in the special issue of the *National Geographic Magazine* telling the story of an Azerbaijani man; Shirali Mislimov. At the age of 167, this guy was still happily working in the fields six days a week and enjoying robust health. Of course, he did eventually die... just shy of his 169th birthday! [9]

No Illness or Disease?

What's just as fascinating about all this is the fact that not only do these cultures live to incredible ages, but illness and disease are virtually non-existent for them.

They don't suffer from deadly diseases like cancer and heart disease.

You won't find any diabetics, nor will you find any people waiting for liver transplants or kidney transplants.

Birth defects are virtually non-existent.

They don't suffer from any of the so-called "degenerative diseases" like we do (osteoporosis, arthritis, Alzheimer's disease, Parkinson's, cataracts, etc).

Women also routinely bear children between the ages of 50 and 60 years. [9]

You won't find any old and decrepit geriatrics stuck in nursing homes either.

What you will find though are people well over the age of a hundred, still enjoying radiant health and vitality and working six to seven days a week.

They don't have any conventional medical doctors because they don't need them! [9]

What Are They Doing That We Aren't?

Obviously, these people must be doing something very right and we must be doing something terribly wrong.

Well, these cultures were studied extensively for over sixty years to find out the reasons why they enjoy such vigorous health and longevity, and here's what was discovered...

The main reason for their long life spans is these people receive, you guessed it, <u>all of the essential nutrients everyday</u> - without them even being aware of it! The main ones of course being minerals and trace elements.

These people live in places where the water they use for irrigation of their food crops is incredibly rich in minerals. This water, known as "glacial milk," comes from under the glaciers in the mountains and contains an abundant supply of all the essential minerals (remember, plants must receive minerals from the soil, they cannot manufacture them).

These people have continued to irrigate their food crops with this water for 2,500 to 5,000 years, *constantly* replenishing the soil with the vital minerals their bodies need. [9,13]

Dr Allen Bannick, who physically went and studied the Hunzas, also observed that when these people finished cooking, they would take the wood ash from their stoves (being a third world country they didn't have access to modern kitchens like we do) and would pour the ash over their vegetable gardens. [10]

Wood ash is nothing but pure minerals!

So naturally, the foods these cultures have been eating for thousands of years have been "mineral rich" foods.

In addition to this, their foods would be incredibly rich in essential vitamins, amino acids and fatty acids – along with life giving chlorophyll - since plants <u>must</u> have minerals in order to make these essential nutrients in high amounts.

More Longevity Secrets...

Along with receiving the vital 90 nutrients we require every day, these people do something else that's been found to be another significant factor in their long life spans.

They practice the art of food fermentation, which in turn, breeds important lactic acid producing bacteria (probiotics). The ingesting of these fermented foods helps to maintain and recolonise a healthy supply of "friendly" bacteria in the digestive system. [16]

Recent health studies have now confirmed that these friendly bacteria do indeed contribute significantly to the overall health and longevity of the human body - much more than what was initially thought (more detailed information on the amazing benefits of good gut bacteria will be provided in Chapter 8).

Once again, these people have been doing something that's crucial to their health for thousands of years, without them even being aware of it.

Actually, the art of food fermentation is nothing new. It's something that's been practised since ancient times, although it's now seriously lacking from our modern day diets.

No Junk Food...

What other factors have been found to contribute to the superior health and longevity these people enjoy?

They don't eat the typical "Western diet" for a start!

Refined and processed foods and junk food aren't a part of their eating regimen (you won't find any Burger King or McDonald's restaurants there, that's for sure).

These people also remain highly active throughout their lives. They continue to do physical work well into their hundreds, and in so doing, keep their bodies (and minds) constantly exercised and stimulated.

We Can all Achieve Longevity

I think the one important thing we all need to keep in mind when it comes to longevity is that it's something which is very achievable for each and every one of us.

Remember, we have the same potential to live to a hundred and beyond as these people do. They aren't "superior beings" to us. They don't have special blood or special cells or anything like that. They are exactly the same as you and I.

We just need to follow their lead and do what they're doing to get the same results… it really is as simple as that!

* * *

I think that if you were unaware of what our genetic potential for longevity was, or that there are indeed certain cultures in the world who enjoy this longevity, then I'm sure you would have found this information as fascinating as I did when I first began researching it.

If you would like to read more about longevity and the long live cultures of the world then I would highly recommend you read the book, Dead Doctors Don't Lie, by Dr Joel Wallach and Dr Ma Lan.

* * *

So now that we have a better understanding of longevity and what's required for us to reach our genetic potential, let's cover these all-important 90 nutrients in more detail.

The next four chapters will be devoted to each of the nutrient categories (minerals, vitamins, amino acids and essential fatty acids) with the succeeding two chapters discussing the benefits of barley grass/live foods and good gut bacteria.

I know that you' re going to find the material contained in these chapters both interesting and informative.

You may even find that some of it might shock you because of what you've been led to believe over the years in regards to your health.

It's time to "separate the wheat from the chaff" though and finally dispel some of the myths and misinformation we've been fed on the subject of nutrition (for example, being told that all fats, including saturated fats, are bad for us, and we can get our daily supply of calcium from milk and other dairy products).

It's all vital information that you'll want to know, and need to know - so let's not delay any more.

Let us begin!

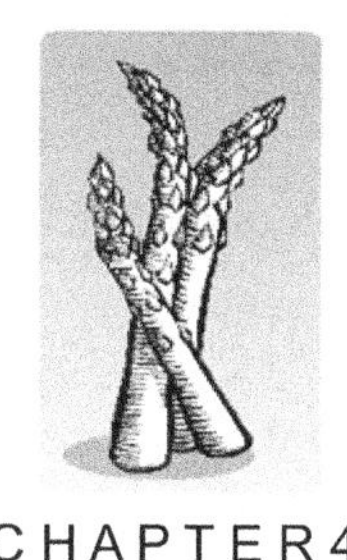

CHAPTER 4

Activate Your Body's Natural (and Potent) Energy Ignighters!

When you look at a breakdown of the 90 nutrients we need every day for optimum health and longevity, you'll notice that two thirds of these nutrients are in fact minerals. We need 60 of them every day, which is a considerable amount. [9]

I would be willing to bet that at least 98% of the population don't receive anywhere close to all 60 a day, let alone in the right proportions. I would also be willing to bet that of the population who *do* receive all 60 everyday, *all* of them would be taking mineral supplements!

When most of us think of nutrition, we tend to think of vitamins not minerals. But we need more than three times the amount of minerals everyday than we do vitamins. They are the bulk of our daily nutritional requirement.

The body can actually manufacture most vitamins. It cannot, however, manufacture minerals in any way, shape or form.

Maintaining Your Chemical Balance is Crucial...

The human body is no different to all of nature. In order for it to survive and flourish it must maintain its proper chemical balance.

This balance is very heavily dependent on the levels and ratios of minerals in the body.

Not only is it imperative that we receive the correct *amount* of minerals every day, the *level* of each mineral is also extremely important.

Each one has an effect on the other, so if one mineral is out of balance, *all* levels will be affected. If this is not corrected, it will cause an array of imbalances that lead to severe fatigue and eventually illness and disease within the body. [13]

In fact, many researchers are now claiming that mineral deficiencies are proving to be the *biggest* cause of lethargy, ill health and premature aging in the world today. And twice Nobel Prize winner and world-renowned doctor, Dr Linus Pauling, once said...

"You can trace every sickness, every disease and every ailment to a mineral deficiency." [8]

That just about covers the whole gamut, doesn't it?

Perfect DNA Synthesis...

One of the most important and crucial functions of the human body is the synthesis of our DNA. For us to remain healthy and active and live to our genetic potential, this process must be carried out everyday in perfect order.

Listen to what biochemist and Medical Research Director for the Longevity Institute of Australia, Bill Anton, says about the importance of minerals in regards to DNA synthesis:

*Minerals play a **critical** role in the synthesis of DNA, which is the* *process of replication and duplication of cell structures. Old cells are constantly being replaced with new cells. This process is almost totally dependent upon trace mineral activity. The body decides how a new cell will be used, and the DNA molecule programs the cell with genetic information so it can function properly. When a cell isn't programmed right because of the lack of essential nutrients it just sits there. It's living, but doesn't know what to do, so it doesn't function. One cell here and there may not matter, but when they accumulate, it's called a tumor, which can result in cancer. When our bodies cannot continuously produce healthy cells, we prematurely age, develop an endless variety of diseases and die before our time.* [13]

So without minerals and trace minerals our health and well-being at the basic cellular level (which is where all life begins and is maintained) becomes severely affected.

Remember this: we are all made up of nothing more than trillions and trillions of individual cells. The health of these individual cells means the health of the whole body.

Why?

Because single cells clump together to form tissues and tissues clump together to form organs - that's how it works. So by keeping all of our individual cells healthy we are in fact keeping our whole body healthy!

Crucial Bodily Functions Requiring Minerals and Trace Minerals...

Aside from cell growth and repair, minerals are needed by the body to build a strong bone structure, for the formation of blood, healthy nerve function, and for building up and maintaining our immune system.

They play an important role in the production and regulation of hormones by the glands (thyroid, parathyroid, ovaries, testes, pancreas, pineal, thymus, adrenals and pituitary) as well as helping us achieve our desired energy levels by activating ATP production. [13,8]

In addition, studies have found that minerals have a very profound effect on the body's enzymes and messenger molecules, which means that without them our bodies wouldn't be able to perform even basic functions such as thinking, breathing, digestion and assimilation! [13]

U.S. Senate Document #264 and *The House Hansard Report...*

So if minerals really are that crucial to our health and longevity, and as a result of the farming methods we use today, all of us are now grossly deficient in these minerals, you may be thinking... "why doesn't our government do something about it then?"

Well, that's a very good question!

And it's not like they haven't known about the problem for some time. The first official warnings were actually reported to the American Government way back in 1936!

In U.S. Senate Document #264 published by the 2nd session of the 74th Congress it was stated:

The alarming fact is that foods – fruits and vegetables and grains, now being raised on millions of acres of land that no longer contain enough of certain needed minerals, are starving us – no matter how much of them we eat. [13,8]

The report went on to say that people who eat these foods develop **mineral deficiency diseases** which can only be corrected by including **mineral supplements** in their diet. It also stated that 99%

of the population is deficient in these minerals, and that a marked deficiency in any one of the more important minerals **actually results in disease**. [13,8]

Can you believe it? They've known about the problem for over 80 years and have done nothing to fix it.

Now I know this report is talking about America, but most Westernized countries have been using the same farming methods for at least the last 80-100 years, so it becomes relevant to everyone.

As a matter of fact, a 1996 Australian Parliamentary report titled *The House Hansard*, paints a similar dire picture. It says:

From preliminary investigations, it has become evident that our soils are equally as deficient in trace minerals as the soils in the United States are (if not more so), not only from the plants' point of view, but also from the human body's point of view.

This report also went on to say:

Without proper mineral balance in our bodies, we cannot function properly and we start degenerating... the sad part is we think it is natural, just a part of getting old. It is not natural and it is not part of getting old. [17]

So let me ask you the obvious question? If it only takes 5-10 years to strip our food crops of all minerals then how depleted do you think they are now?

Is it just a coincidence that we have mineral deficient soils and we now have one of the worst disease and early death rates in the world?

I would actually go as far as to say that the decline in health of the human race over the past 10 years has now hit catastrophic levels.

At the time of writing this book, a close family friend recently passed away from cancer. A work colleague also just lost his father-in-law to cancer, and two other friends have fathers who have terminal cancer. Another colleague died recently of a heart attack.

And these are only people I know!

They are (or were) all under the age of 65 too, by the way.

It's like we're dropping like flies!

Now what really concerns me about the U.S. Senate report and the Australian Parliamentary report is not just the fact that nothing has been done to address the problem, but the fact that we have been (and still are being) deceived into believing that we can obtain all the nutrients we need from our diet.

What an absolute load of rubbish!

If something is not done about this problem then millions of people are going to continue to die prematurely, and in my opinion, totally unnecessarily!

Minerals and Their Key Functions...

Okay, now that I've got that off my chest, let's have a look at some of the more common minerals we need everyday and see exactly how they benefit us, along with what illnesses and diseases they can prevent and even treat.

Nutritionally speaking, there are two groups of minerals we need to be concerned with...

The first group is the macrominerals or bulk minerals, and these include calcium, sodium, phosphorus, magnesium and potassium.

These minerals are needed in fairly large quantities.

The second group are microminerals or trace minerals, and these include boron, chromium, iodine, copper, iron, selenium, zinc, manganese, vanadium and cobalt. These minerals are needed in smaller quantities but are nonetheless just as important as the macrominerals. [13]

Calcium...

Calcium is probably the one mineral that virtually everyone has heard of. We know that we need it to build strong teeth and bones, however, this is not its only function.

Calcium is also crucial for cardiovascular function and for regulating our heartbeat. Without it our bodies cannot maintain their correct acid/alkaline balance, which in turn leads to a variety of health problems and diseases including cancer.

<u>Calcium is such an essential nutrient that a deficiency can actually cause over 147 different diseases in the body!</u> [9]

Quite amazing don't you think?

And because the body requires a sufficient supply of *absorbable* calcium every day, if it doesn't get what it needs it will basically "eat up" its own bones in order to make up the deficit.

What's interesting about this though is if you were to test the blood of a person with a serious calcium deficiency you would actually find it to be at the normal physiological levels.

Why is this?

Because the parathyroid glands will literally *force* the body to take calcium from the bones as long as it has to in order to maintain the critical balance needed in the blood (a process called *homeostasis*.)[13]

So even though the test would show the person has normal levels of calcium in the blood, he or she would in fact be seriously depleted.

The body would eventually drain the bones so low that calcium deficient diseases such as osteoporosis and arthritis would prevail. (When the bones become severely depleted of calcium they can actually turn as soft as frozen ice cream). [13]

We used to only see problems such as arthritis and soft bone fractures in the elderly, but now children are also being affected as a result of calcium deficiencies.

That tells you how bad the problem has become.

You Need Trace Minerals for Calcium Absorption

When it comes to calcium absorption, trace minerals are an essential component as the body is unable to assimilate this nutrient (or any nutrient, for that matter) on its own.

An experiment that was done with women suffering from osteoporosis verifies this...

The women were divided into three groups. The first group received a placebo. The second group received high doses of calcium. The third group received calcium plus trace minerals (magnesium, copper, zinc, manganese, boron etc.). After two years of the experiment the women were re-tested for bone thickness. The first group, the placebo group, had a *marked decrease* in bone thickness. The second group, who received high doses of calcium, had a *moderate decrease* in bone thickness. The third group, who received calcium plus trace minerals, had a *marked increase* in bone thickness. [1]

Stay Away From Daisy...

Of course, we're constantly being informed by various advertisements on the TV, radio and internet that we need to consume milk and other dairy products to get our daily supply of calcium.

Well, here's a question...

If this is true then why is it that the U.S., Australia and New Zealand - three of the largest dairy consuming nations per capita in the world - have the highest rates of osteoporosis in the world? Many Asian countries do not consume milk yet have low rates of osteoporosis? [13]

The reason for this is the calcium contained in milk is very difficult for the body to assimilate, even if you drink cartons of it (and regardless if it's fortified with extra calcium).

Dairy products are simply not the answer to a calcium deficiency.

On the other hand, the calcium that's contained in wheat grass and colloidal minerals is 98% absorbable. This is the right kind of calcium your body needs! [9]

Diseases and Ailments Caused by a Calcium Deficiency...

a. Osteoporosis (porous bones). This is the major one. Caused when the bones are continuously leached of calcium by the parathyroid glands. Osteoporosis results in brittle bones that fracture very easily. [1,13]

b. Receding gums and gingivitis. These are caused by osteoporosis of the jawbones and facial bones. Although brushing your teeth daily is important, this is actually not the main cause of these two problems. [1]

c. Lower back pain. This is caused by osteoporosis of the vertebrae. As the bones in the vertebrae become soft and brittle, they continue to wear down causing pain and inflammation. [1]

d. Arthritis. 85% of all arthritis is caused by osteoporosis of the joint ends of the bones. If you suffer from arthritis then taking in a daily supply of colloidal minerals and organic wheat grass powder is an absolute must. Not only do you need calcium, but also boron (crucial), magnesium, zinc, selenium, copper, iron and manganese, along with the B group vitamins and vitamins D, C and E, which are all extremely important for bone health. [1,3,13]

And while we're on the subject of arthritis, various studies have now been able to prove that two substances, glucosamine and chondroitin, can help arthritis sufferers tremendously. Both substances are natural and safe. The glucosamine sulphate helps arthritic joints by actually rebuilding cartilage and bone matrix (something that up until recently was thought could not occur). The chondroitin then attracts fluid into the joints to help maintain lubrication. Numerous tests that have been carried out on patients suffering from osteoarthritis have produced some outstanding results. Most report excellent improvement in joint mobility and "overwhelming" relief from their pain and inflammation. [18]

Funnily enough, the original discovery of glucosamine and chrondroitin stemmed from a published study carried out by Harvard Medical School (and aptly titled, *Chicken Protein Halts the Swelling and Pain of Arthritis)...*

In a patient trial, 29 volunteers who failed to respond to medical treatments for their arthritis were given a heaped teaspoon of grounded up chicken cartilage in their orange juice every morning.

According to research organizers, within 3 months all participants reported improved joint mobility and within 6 months their pain and inflammation had disappeared! [14]

If you're interested, glucosamine and chrondroitin supplements combined with MSM (for extra benefit), are available from most health food stores or online and are reasonably priced. If you cannot afford to buy these then having a teaspoonful of Gelatine everyday can help (having all of them together works even better). Gelatine is also made from the same raw material as our own cartilage. Keep in mind that results will *only* be positive and maximised when these are taken in combination with *all* of the 90 essential nutrients.

e. Kidney stones. Here's one health problem that has been completely misdiagnosed for years. Doctors used to think that kidney stones were the result of having too much calcium in the body. So what they would do is tell their patients to cut out all foods that contain calcium from their diet. Thankfully, we now know that kidney stones are <u>not</u> the result of having too much calcium, instead, they actually come from your <u>own</u> bones when you have a raging calcium deficiency! [1,13]

Remember earlier I said that if the body doesn't receive enough calcium from the diet, it will take what it needs from the bones? Well, kidney stones are the result of this. These "stones" are nothing more than crystallised deposits of calcium that have come from the bones. [1,13]

An article from Harvard Medical School published back in March of 1993 confirms this. The article titled *Calcium Limits Kidney Stone Risk* stated:

In a study that turns conventional medical wisdom on its head, researchers have found that people whose diets are rich in calcium run a reduced risk of developing kidney stones. In a study of more than 45,000 people who were ranked into five categories, the group that received the most calcium had no kidney stones. [1]

f. Bone spurs/heel spurs. Bone spurs are affecting more and more people today. As the body continues to pull calcium from the bones (as a result of a deficiency), they naturally become soft and brittle and bone spurs occur.

If you've ever had bone spurs, you'll notice they usually form where the tendons attach to bone. Whenever the tendon is used it pulls a spur causing considerable pain. Bone spurs are a good indication of a serious calcium deficiency. [1,13]

g. *High blood pressure*. How many times have you heard that an excessive amount of salt intake will cause high blood pressure? Well, a 20 year study conducted on salt and HBP has now proven otherwise...

In the first part of the study, 5,000 people who suffered from acute high blood pressure were taken off their medication and placed on a full salt restricted diet.

All of them died!

In the second part of the study another 5,000 people with HBP were once again taken off their medication, but this time were given calcium supplements at double the recommended daily allowance and no salt restriction. After 6 weeks the experiment was stopped as 85% of participants were cured of their high blood pressure. [1]

And back in July of 1997, the American Heart Association came out with an interesting article titled *Doctors Lack Proof that too Much Salt is bad for you*. It said that *"after years of telling healthy people that too much salt isn't good for them, researchers still don't have solid evidence to back up that claim."* [19]

Further extensive studies on salt and high blood pressure carried out by cardiologist, Dr Alexander Gordon Logan, have also confirmed that restricting salt does not prevent or lower high blood pressure one bit! [19]

So along with keeping my calcium intake up, I now go ahead and salt all my food to taste without feeling guilty (using healthy salt options such as Himalayan pink rock salt or Celtic Sea salt).

I suggest you do the same!

Other ailments caused from a calcium deficiency include: gout, insomnia, P.M.S, dental cavities, irritability, leg or menstrual cramps, sore/aching joints, spinal curvature, Paget's disease, sore tendons and bursitis. [13]

Selenium...

As one of the more recently discovered minerals, selenium's importance is just now becoming recognized.

It's been hailed as one of the finest and most powerful antioxidants available and plays a vital role in the detoxification process - which in turn protects the body's cells and promotes a longer life span. [1]

Selenium is also known as the "anti-cancer mineral" and has been shown in studies to prevent chromosome mutations. This means cells are unable to multiply unrestrained and turn cancerous. The British Medical Journal confirms this by reporting that the use of selenium supplements on patients cut cancer rates by half. [8]

Back in December of 1996, the University of Arizona Medical School published the results of a randomized, placebo-controlled, double blind study on cancer and selenium headed by Dr Larry C. Clarke:

In the study, three hundred people were given 200 micrograms of selenium daily, then watched closely for ten years. What researchers uncovered was amazing...

They found that selenium was able to reduce oesophageal cancer in all participants by 71%. It was able to reduce prostate cancer in men by 69%. It was able to reduce colon and rectal cancers by 62%. It was able to reduce lung cancer by 48%, whether they were smokers or not. And in a parallel study conducted by the University of California San Diego, researchers discovered that selenium was able to reduce breast cancer in women by 65-95%, depending on the type. [19]

Wow!

Now the FDA actually recognizes selenium as an *anti-cancer nutrient*. [20]

Selenium for a Healthy Heart

A selenium deficiency has also been linked to a lot of heart problems. In fact, this mineral is well known to *prevent* cardiomyopathy (a heart degeneration disease) by strengthening and protecting the heart muscle.

It's been discovered in Finland - where they have excessively high rates of heart disease - they have low intakes of selenium. And in parts of China, a disease known as Keshan disease (which causes heart failure) has also been found to be the result of a selenium deficiency. [1,8,20]

So evidence is now beginning to show just how crucial this mineral is in the prevention and cure of the world's two biggest killers. A leading editorial article from the British Medical Journal adds weight to this by saying: *"The low bio-availability of selenium could be contributing to cancers and heart disease world wide."* [8]

More Powerful Health Benefits of Selenium...

What else do we need selenium for?

It's essential for healthy reproductive functions (in both men and women) and for the production of thyroid hormones. It also boosts and strengthens the immune system significantly by increasing antibody production, along with helping to protect the joints from the symptoms of rheumatoid arthritis.

In laboratory studies, selenium has been shown to halt liver damage (cirrhosis) as well as regenerate the liver. It's also an accepted remedy for acute pancreatitis, septicemia and Lymphedema (when the lymph nodes have been removed due to breast cancer). [20]

One of the top 10 most quoted scientists in the world and selenium expert, Dr Gerhard Schrauzer, recommends selenium for HIV positive patients.

He and his colleagues have seen outstanding results with selenium in the treatment of the AIDS virus - which they believe is due to its ability to halt harmful oxygen radical production in the body. Dr Schrauzer also discovered that taking high doses of selenium helps to reduce the neurological damage in the brain caused by strokes.

Further studies have shown that low selenium levels cause severe depression and mood swings and high levels produce improved eyesight, improved brain function and heightened moods. [13,20]

Other diseases and ailments caused from a selenium deficiency include: birth defects, SIDS, anaemia, impotence, infertility, brain problems, candida (thrush), chronic fatigue syndrome, cystic fibrosis, multiple sclerosis, muscular dystrophy and cataracts. [13]

Copper...

Like selenium, copper is known as an "anti-cancer" and "anti-carcinogenic" mineral.

What's just as fascinating about copper is not only does it help prevent cancers from forming, it can also treat the disease. [8]

And because copper is anti-carcinogenic, it's a powerful antioxidant that helps protect against harmful free radical or oxygen radical damage (for a detailed explanation on free radicals and antioxidants and how they affect our health, see Chapter 8 titled "*Wheat Grass*… Nature's Astonishing Miracle Food").

Copper is also important for bone health and a deficiency will result in osteoporosis, arthritis and an increased rate of bone fractures.[8]

It's necessary for healthy brain nerves and for the forming of connective tissues. A deficiency will also cause heart disease, anaemia and a low white blood cell count, which means it then becomes increasingly difficult for the body to fight off infection and disease.[13]

Copper Prevents Aneurysms...

Another important benefit of copper is that it's known to prevent ruptured aneurysms (the ballooning and bursting of an artery).[1]

Aneurysms are yet another health problem that have become rampant amongst society today, although we don't hear much about them. They can occur anywhere in the body but the main type is a ruptured aortic aneurysm (the aorta is the main artery from the heart). When this happens, the person will usually be deceased before they hit the ground.

Other common aneurysms occur in the brain and can cause everything from stroke-like damage (paralysis, etc.) to death.

One autopsy study revealed that 40% – just under half of all people examined – who died of other causes, actually had aneurysms somewhere in their bodies.

In a separate study, a physician was able to measure the copper levels in the arterial walls of patients who had ruptured aortic aneurysms. They were found to be 75% lower than normal.[8]

Other research has found that the plak (a cholesterol/calcium complex that forms in the arterial walls of heart disease patients) contains very low levels of copper. This substance, which actually forms as a result of small cracks in the arteries (the body uses the plak to try and plug up these holes), only appears in the first place because of an elastic fibre breakdown due to a <u>severe</u> copper deficiency! [8,21]

Further studies done on animals such as turkeys have also been able to confirm just how much of a vital role copper does play in the prevention of aneurysms.[1]

Signs of a Copper Deficiency

So what are some of the obvious signs of a copper deficiency?

Well, the first one to look for is greying hair, no matter your age. Contrary to popular belief, grey hair is *not* hereditary. It's caused by low levels of copper.

And the greyer the hair the worse the problem!

If you've ever seen photos of Albert Einstein not long before he died, you'll instantly recognize his bright grey hair. Einstein died of a ruptured aneurysm – a simple copper deficiency.

So if you do have grey hair then start taking in a daily supply of colloidal minerals, colloidal copper, and organic mineral rich wheat grass powder and watch your hair "magically" return to its natural colour within 8-12 months. And remember this; if the bad stuff's going away on the outside, it's going away on the inside as well!

Some other signs of a copper deficiency include; skin wrinkles and crow's feet around the eyes (elastic fibre breakdown) and sagging skin around the arms, breasts, neck, stomach and legs (also the result of an elastic fibre breakdown).[1,13]

Other diseases and ailments caused from a copper deficiency include: liver cirrhosis and dysfunction, birth defects, infertility, iron storage disease and depression. [9,13]

Zinc...

Known as the "superstar" mineral, zinc can be found in virtually every tissue of the body. Research has not only shown it to be one of the more important minerals, but that nearly everyone is grossly deficient in it.

One of the major benefits found with zinc is its ability to prevent and even treat one of the biggest killers in men today... prostate cancer. [21]

Further research has shown that it plays a crucial role in the prevention and treatment of infertility problems and protecting unborn babies from birth defects. [22]

Zinc is needed for the action and production of several hormones including insulin, growth hormone, testosterone and estrogen. In fact, with regards to insulin, zinc plays such an essential role in regulating insulin activity that it's now considered one of *the* most important nutrients for *all* diabetics and pre-diabetic patients. [13,23]

More Reasons to Get Your Zinc Every Day...

Zinc is a required nutrient for DNA synthesis and for the maintenance and building of a strong immune system. It's well known for its ability to not only prevent the onset of dreaded cold and flu viruses (influenza), but also reduce the severity if one does become exposed to these.

In addition, zinc has been found to be an essential part of a wide range of enzymes (these are protein structures that are crucial for all bodily functions). Zinc is involved in over 250 enzyme systems, including one very important enzyme known as super oxide dismutase (which will be explained in detail in Chapter 8). [13,23]

Zinc is also needed for strong bone growth and for the healthy healing of wounds. It helps with maintaining the health of the eyes and is useful in preventing and treating certain skin disorders such as acne. A deficiency has been linked to cystic fibrosis, along with other problems such as retarded growth and impaired sexual function. [13,23]

Other symptoms of a zinc deficiency include: asthma, slow healing of wounds, poor sense of taste and smell, lethargy, skin lesions, brittle hair and nails, hyperactivity, candida, chronic fatigue syndrome, PMS and diabetes. [13,23]

(*Note*: one of the first signs of a zinc deficiency is white flakes under the fingernails. If you find you have these then be sure to get some colloidal zinc into you... fast!).

Chromium/Vanadium...

These two minerals are rapidly gaining recognition as to their significant importance to our health, *especially* in regards to preventing and treating diabetes. As a matter of fact, studies have now been able to prove that a chromium deficiency, if left for too long, will actually result in the onset of diabetes! [1]

How Exactly Do They Help?

Chromium is part of what's known as "Glucose Tolerance

Factor". When it's combined with vanadium, it's able to regulate blood sugar levels and cholesterol. So if a person's blood sugar is too low, it will regulate it up, and if it's too high it will regulate it down.[1]

What this means is these two minerals will regulate normal insulin activity in the body, and in turn, control hypoglycemia and adult-onset diabetes.

The University of Vancouver School of Medicine in British Columbia actually stated that: "V*anadium alone will replace insulin in adult onset diabetics.*" And an intensive study that was subsequently conducted by the same University on insulin dependent diabetics using vanadium in place of insulin verified this statement. [1,13]

Heart Disease and Cancer Protectors

Chromium and vanadium are also important for the heart and play a powerful role in protecting the body against heart disease and cancer (yet another nutrient(s) that help in the fight against the world's two biggest killers).

Chromium in particular is essential for the metabolism of cholesterol and fats in the blood, and because of this, helps to prevent atherosclerosis or "hardening of the arteries". [13]

A recent medical article reiterates this by saying...

Chromium depletion coupled with diets high in refined carbohydrates can cause glucose intolerance and increased insulin and fat levels in the blood. These metabolic disturbances could explain why atherosclerosis (hardening of the arteries) is so common in most Western societies. [8]

Other diseases and ailments caused from a chromium and/or vanadium deficiency include: hyperactivity, immune weakness, impotence, infertility, candida, chronic fatigue syndrome, kidney failure, digestive problems, depression and PMS. [13]

Magnesium...

Magnesium is one of the main necessary elements of nerve fibres and a deficiency is known to cause cramp and spasm problems. It comes as no surprise then that a magnesium deficiency is also the leading cause of serious nerve disorders such as convulsive fits, epilepsy and seizures. [13]

Other types of cramps and spasms including muscular twitching and menstrual pain are also the result of a lack of magnesium, along with any shooting, stabbing or irregular pain such as angina, sciatica, neuritis, neuralgia, and some types of migraine headaches.[3,13]

Another Heart Protector

Research has found that magnesium goes hand in hand with chromium in being essential for the health of the heart and preventing the build-up of cholesterol in the arteries.

In fact, a magnesium deficiency, without any prior warning, can cause serious heart problems such as cardiac arrhythmia (sudden cardiac death), cardiac disease and heart attack!

Approximately three hundred thousand cardiac deaths each year are actually linked to a magnesium deficiency. [13]

A study performed back in 1957 on magnesium therapy versus anticoagulant drugs in helping patients with coronary thrombosis (a blood clot in the coronary artery) validates the importance of magnesium in the prevention and treatment of heart problems...

In a one-year period, 196 patients suffering severe coronary heart disease were treated with normally prescribed anticoagulant drugs.

60 of these patients died.

The following year 100 patients suffering similar coronary complaints were treated with parenterally administered magnesium.

Remarkably, only 1 died!

This ground-breaking study was first published in the *British Medical Journal* back in January 1960. [13]

Magnesium for Bone Health

70% of magnesium is located in the bones and teeth, along with calcium and phosphorus, which makes it an important nutrient for the healthy growth and maintenance of teeth and bones.

It's also needed for calcium and potassium absorption, balancing the body's pH levels, ATP production and utilization, and for the burning of glycogen (carbohydrates) for fuel. [3,13]

Other diseases and problems caused by a magnesium deficiency include: kidney stones, hyperactivity, arthritis, osteoporosis, hypothermia, constipation, birth defects, premature aging, nervousness and receding gums. [3,13]

Iron...

This mineral is present in every human cell and is a vital component of blood.

It's involved in the formation of hemoglobin – the essential part of red blood cells. Hemoglobin is necessary for the transportation of oxygen from the lungs to the cells, along with the removing of carbon dioxide from the cells to be transported back to the lungs (to then be expelled).

An iron deficiency means this process is unable to be accomplished efficiently so unwanted health problems then result; the major one being anemia.

When this happens the capacity for the body to carry oxygen and produce energy is greatly diminished, which in turn causes fatigue, lack of energy and shortness of breath.[3,23]

The most obvious sign of anemia is severe paleness of the skin.

More Benefits of Iron...

Iron helps with the synthesis of collagen, which is essential for healthy teeth, gums, cartilage and bones. It assists with one's ability to concentrate and with memory recall, along with helping the body build resistance to emotional stress, infections and disease through increased antibody production.

The enzymes that are needed for the synthesis of DNA and RNA cannot function correctly without an adequate supply of daily iron. [3,23]

Other diseases and ailments caused by an iron deficiency include: asthma, constipation, depression, acute infections, colds and flu, dizziness and headaches. [3,23]

Boron...

One of boron's main functions is to keep calcium in the bones. This makes it a crucial nutrient for bone health and for the prevention and treatment of bone degeneration diseases such as osteoporosis and arthritis.

Boron is also important for the manufacture of hormones, and although it does help men make testosterone, it doesn't increase their levels above normal, nor is it "anabolic" and able to stimulate muscle growth (as some supplement companies claim).

In women, boron acts similar to estrogen and a deficiency will cause females to suffer badly through menopause.

A boron deficiency is also known to affect the brain and kidneys, along with being a major contributing factor in teeth and gum problems including receding gums and gingivitis.[1,8,13]

Other diseases and ailments caused by a boron deficiency include: arteriosclerosis, cancer (especially breast and prostate), kidney stones, gout, juvenile arthritis, lupus, psoriasis, eczema, fibromyalgia, rosacea, back pain, bone spurs, erectile dysfunction, candida and yeast fungus (thrush).

Where Do You Get Your Boron From?

Boron is just one of the many important minerals we need everyday that you won't find in most multi-vitamin and mineral supplements (I've only managed to find a couple that contain it). As I said, one of boron's main functions is to keep calcium in the bones yet virtually none of the calcium supplements on the market contain any boron!

Thankfully, it is found in liquid colloidal minerals and organic wheat grass supplements, although the best (and cheapest) source is actually Borax. Yes I know, this sounds ridiculous but I strongly suggest you take the time to search online and read the article titled

"The Borax Conspiracy – How the Arthritis Cure Has Been Stopped" by Walter Last.

You'll definitely change your mind about Borax after reading this!

Manganese...

Manganese plays a crucial role in the digestion and utilisation of fats and the controlling of cholesterol in the blood. It's important for insulin production and is known to lessen the severity of diabetes mellitus.

It's also needed for correct co-ordination between the brain, nerves and muscles, and because of this, a deficiency has been linked to nerve disorders such as convulsions, seizures, epilepsy, and Multiple Sclerosis. [8,13]

Manganese makes up part of the body's own antioxidant system (super oxide dismutase) which protects the cells against free radical damage. It's an essential nutrient for thyroid and sex hormone production, as well as for the healthy functioning of the mammary glands.

More Benefits of Manganese...

Manganese is important to expectant mothers as it's associated with the "maternal instinct" and is necessary for the healthy nerve, skeletal and brain development of their unborn child. [3,13,23]

Manganese is also vital for the formation of bone, collagen and connective tissue and forms a part of what's known as prothrombin for blood clotting. A deficiency can cause problems such as retarded growth, male and female sterility, impotence and digestive troubles.[3,13,23]

Other diseases and problems caused by a manganese deficiency include: memory loss, cystic fibrosis, asthma, birth defects, impaired hearing or deafness, poor coordination and abnormal bone development.[3,23]

Germanium...

This mineral has become "big news" as far as scientific discoveries go. Research has shown that germanium plays a key role in protecting the body against *all* forms of cancer and heart related diseases.

Many doctors in Japan, Austria, Germany and Poland have been using germanium for the past thirty years to treat cancer, osteoporosis and rheumatoid arthritis... with outstanding results. In fact, the success rate has been so high that some clinics in Japan won't use anything else! [3]

Germanium is also known to greatly improve oxygen supply to the body along with boosting the immune system. This in turn helps with a more rapid recovery from illness and many of the chronic ailments that plague society today.

Most of us know about the amazing healing properties of aloe vera, ginseng and garlic. Well, germanium is believed to be the main healing component of these three plants! [3]

Potassium...

Potassium is required for the correct functioning of the cells, nerves and muscles. It combines with sodium to help maintain the right fluid and electrolyte balances in the tissues and cells.

In particular, potassium maintains the correct acid/alkaline balance in the digestive system, resulting in better digestion and assimilation of food, along with the prevention of hyper-acidity problems such as heartburn and acid reflux (GERD). [3,13]

Potassium is also needed for hormone production, regulating blood pressure and for correct heart functioning. Labelled "detergent for the arteries," it's particularly effective for cleaning and flushing out the plak from arteries and arterial walls (reversing arteriosclerosis). [2]

A potassium deficiency is known to cause problems such as edema (fluid retention), gastro-intestinal disorders, fatigue, depression and nervous disorders. [3,13]

Other diseases and ailments caused by a potassium deficiency include: cystic fibrosis, multiple sclerosis, constipation, receding gums, muscular weakness, irritability and mental exhaustion. [3,13]

Lithium...

This is yet another mineral that helps in the prevention and treatment of heart disease (there's getting to be a few, isn't there?). Recent studies have found that patients who suffer from heart disease have very low levels of lithium in their bodies.[8]

Lithium is also known to treat the manic stage of the manic-depressive, along with a condition known as Meniere's disease (an ailment of the inner ear characterized by vertigo, tinnitus and hearing loss). [24]

Further studies have confirmed that a lithium deficiency can cause learning disabilities, hyperactivity, and even criminal behaviour. Tests carried out on violent criminals have shown their bodies contain extremely low levels of lithium.

A close link between ADHD and a lithium deficiency has also recently been discovered. [8,24]

Iodine...

Iodine is very important for the healthy functioning and maintenance of the thyroid gland. It's needed for the manufacturing of our thyroid hormones, which in turn regulate our physical and mental development, cellular metabolism and energy production.[3,23]

When someone is suffering from constant physical or mental fatigue or a sluggish metabolism, one of the first causes is often a problem with their thyroid gland. This can usually be remedied by taking in some supplemental iodine.

The most common problems caused by an iodine deficiency include goitre (enlargement of the thyroid gland), birth defects (such as mental retardation), lethargy and being unable to keep excess weight off. A serious iodine deficiency can result in thyroid cancer, high cholesterol and heart disease. [3,23]

Other ailments caused by an iodine deficiency include: stunted growth, rough and wrinkled skin, low blood pressure and anemia. [3,23]

Silica...

Silica is often referred to as the "beauty mineral" as it forms part of collagen - the substance that joins cells together. It's needed for the proper elasticity of human tissue, particularly skin tissue, so it naturally helps prevent wrinkles and sagging skin from forming.[3]

Silica is known to aid in bone formation and assist with the healing of torn ligaments and tendons. It's important for the health of the hair and nails, as well as being a powerful cleanser and eliminator. Silica has also been found to be beneficial in the healing of boils, abscesses, styes, and arthritic calcium spurs. [3]

Sodium...

Sodium, along with potassium and chloride, is one of the body's three main electrolytes. These key minerals perform a variety of essential functions including regulating the balance of body fluids and regulating nerve and muscle function. Sodium is in fact largely responsible for controlling the body's *total* water content. [13]

Because sodium (salt) is added to just about every type of processed food, most people already receive plenty. The problem though is this is usually the *wrong* type of sodium!

Make sure your sodium <u>only</u> comes from healthy sources such as Himalayan pink rock salt or Celtic Sea salt. Remember too that athletes need more sodium, especially when exercising in warmer weather.

Phosphorus...

This mineral combines with calcium to build strong bones and teeth. However, phosphorus can cause reduced calcium absorption and calcium loss from the bones and teeth if there's too much in the diet, so you do need to be careful.

Unfortunately, we're now seeing a serious "phosphorous overload" occurring as a result of this mineral being added to cola-type drinks, soft drinks, energy drinks and many refined and processed foods. Consuming these products greatly increases the risk of you developing diseases like osteoporosis and arthritis, along with suffering teeth and gum problems such as tooth decay and gingivitis. [3,12]

So the best way to avoid this from happening is of course to cut out, or at the very least, seriously limit the amount of soft drinks and refined and processed foods in your diet. These foods are usually low in calcium and high in phosphorus, which results in a calcium-phosphorus imbalance.

The fruits and vegetables you buy from the supermarket also contain high amounts of phosphorous from the overuse of NPK fertilizers so a deficiency of this nutrient is rare. [3,12]

Other Important Minerals...

Tin is one mineral that is vital for hair growth and preventing male pattern baldness.

Molybdenum is involved in the manufacture of DNA and RNA and has just recently been discovered in tooth enamel, suggesting it may help in the prevention of tooth decay.

Galleon has been shown in studies to reduce cancer in children.

Then there's another group of seven minerals known as "rare earths" which when given to laboratory animals, doubled their lifespan! [1,23]

Silver, Nickel and Arsenic...

So the list of essential minerals continues on.

Remember, they're all critically important to our health and longevity and each one has a very distinctive and crucial role to play – even trace minerals such as silver, nickel and arsenic.

In fact, arsenic was used in a study back in the 1970's for the treatment of cancer that was actually labelled "so crazy and ridiculous it couldn't possibly work"...

Scientists took 15 patients who were suffering from Acute Promyelocytic Leukemia or APL (one of the most aggressive forms of cancers) and gave them 15 milligrams of arsenic trioxide intravenously each day.

Now, keep in mind that when someone gets this disease it's usually considered a death sentence as most patients die within the first 3 months of diagnosis.

Well, after 3 months, 8 people went into remission, and remarkably, after a year *all* of the participants were considered "cured!" [19]

This powerful finding, along with other subsequent studies and reviewed data on the benefits of arsenic for APL, were later confirmed by world-renowned cancer and leukemia expert, Dr. Meir Wetzler. As a result of this, arsenic trioxide has now become part of the standard care for patients with APL! [53]

Supplementation...

So as I said at the beginning of this chapter, we each need 60 minerals every day, and as you've no doubt gathered by now, we aren't going to get them from our diet.

So how do we?

Simple... supplementation, which is an absolute ***must!***

There are basically three ways for us to do this...

The first way is to consume what are known as metallic minerals. These are essentially just powdered rock. Metallic minerals are only about 8-12% absorbable by the body.

Unfortunately, many of the vitamin and mineral supplements on the market today contain metallic minerals (because they're cheap to source and manufacture).

The body really does have a difficult time trying to digest these types of minerals. They can actually pass straight through the digestive tract totally undissolved! Metallic minerals can also be toxic to the body in large amounts and can cause constipation.

The second way that we can take in the minerals we need is by consuming what are known as chelated minerals. This means the minerals are bonded to protein molecules. These molecules are what transport the minerals into the bloodstream, thereby enhancing their absorption rate.

Chelated minerals are estimated to be around 40% absorbable. [1]

Many of the more reputable multi-vitamin and mineral supplements on the market contain chelated minerals.

The third and most *efficient* way to consume the minerals we need is in the plant based colloidal form.

Plant based colloidal minerals are about 98% absorbable.

Most formulations also contain all 60 minerals (and even up to 75), whereas the synthetic multi-vitamin and mineral supplements only contain around 10-14 (where are the other 46 or more minerals?).

Plant based colloidal minerals are also not toxic to the body in any way, even though they contain minerals such as lead and arsenic (of course our bodies need these minerals in trace amounts). [1,13]

You may remember at the start of this chapter I explained how the body *must* receive minerals in the correct amounts and ratios for complete absorption?

Well, this is simply not possible when consuming multi-vitamin and mineral tablets or formulas. This **is** possible though when you consume plant based colloidal minerals!

The way it works is like this... Plants take metallic minerals from out of the ground and absorb them up through their root system. Then, by the process of photosynthesis, alter the structure of the mineral so it becomes "organic." The human body is now able to recognize, assimilate, and more importantly, utilize these organic compounds (minerals) for its own benefit.

This is the way our bodies are designed to absorb minerals – in the organic, plant based form. There is another (complimentary) way to get the minerals you need as well... by consuming Himalayan pink rock salt or Celtic Sea salt (which both contain over 84 minerals and trace elements in a highly absorbable form). I'll be explaining more about these in an upcoming chapter. [1,13]

Because plant based colloidal minerals are still a relatively new type of supplement on the market, you need to make sure that what you buy contains what it's supposed to – at least 60 minerals.

I believe a plant based colloidal mineral supplement that contains Moorlife minerals or minerals from the humic shale deposit would be a very good and wise choice.

* * *

That ends this chapter on minerals.

Hopefully, you now have a better understanding as to **why** we need these powerful little "super chargers" so badly.

Another type of nutrient(s) we need every day is vitamins, which also have a significant role to play in our health and longevity program.

Let's find out why...

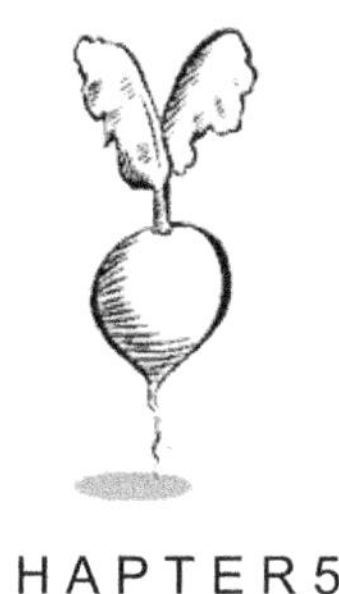

16 Powerful Nutrients for Health and Vitality...

The medical field has regarded the discovery of vitamins as one of the most important nutritional discoveries of the 20th century.

Now, that's a pretty big statement, but certainly a worthy one.

It was once thought that illness and disease could only occur through the action of certain agents such as bacteria. However, when vitamins were discovered, scientists realized that disease and illness could arise from a *lack* of something, or more specifically, the absence of certain organic compounds in the diet. Once verified, these organic compounds were then considered *essential* for good health and longevity. [3,23]

It's now been firmly established that vitamins not only perform several specific and key functions, they also prevent and treat a wide range of deficiency diseases.

Even though the body can manufacture many of the vitamins we need, one must not make the mistake of believing that we don't need a daily supply from our diet.

Factors such as pollution, poor eating habits and a lack of the other available nutrients in our foods all mean the body requires a greater supply than it's able to provide for itself.

As we age, it then becomes more and more difficult for the body to manufacture vitamins - so making sure we obtain these from our diet as we grow older takes on even more importance.

In addition to this, without the correct amounts and ratios of vitamin intake every day over a thousand chemical and enzymatic processes in the body are severely affected and weakened over time. What this means in layman's terms is your susceptibility to disease and ill health increases considerably! [3,23]

A little while back, *Time* magazine ran a terrific article titled *The Real Power of Vitamins*. One of the key headlines in that write-up said it all... *"Research Shows They May Help Fight Cancer, Heart Disease and the Ravages of Ageing."* [18]

And the World Health Organization (WHO) once made this bold statement... *"Vitamins can help two billion children."* Considering there's only 2.2 billion kids on the planet, that's a pretty substantial amount! [18]

Go Natural...

As with the other nutrients we need, our bodies are incapable of absorbing vitamins on their own. Minerals and live enzymes, along with amino acids, are needed for any vitamin to be assimilated and utilized correctly. For example, vitamin E cannot be absorbed without correct levels of colloidal zinc in the blood. [13]

For this reason, vitamins must come from natural food sources rather than synthetic vitamin tablets or formulas. The synthetic versions never produce the same effect as vitamins that are still in their pure and natural form (they do make your urine turn a lovely bright yellow color though!).

When it comes to vitamins, most people are unaware of the

crucial role minerals actually play in the body's use of vitamins (yes, I know I'm back onto minerals again, but with good reason).

An extract from U.S. Senate Document #264 explains this. It reads:

We know that vitamins are complex chemical substances which are indispensable to nutrition, and that each of them is of importance for the normal function of some special structure of the body. Disorder and disease result from any vitamin deficiency. It is not commonly realised, however, that vitamins control the body's appropriation of minerals, and in the absence of minerals, they have no function to perform. Lacking vitamins, the system can make some use of minerals; but lacking minerals, vitamins are useless.[13]

So, without minerals, vitamins are useless?

This means you can go and pop all the vitamin pills you want, but unless you have minerals to go with them, you're just wasting your money and not gaining any health benefits.

That's why supplementing our diets with nutrient rich foods such as organic wheat grass or barley grass is so important as these contain the full spectrum of vitamins, along with minerals, amino acids and valuable live enzymes for absorption!

Vitamins and Their Functions...

Let's now have a look at some of the more important vitamins we need every day, along with some of the reasons *why* we need them, and some of the key functions they perform. (Note: Because vitamins tie in with the body's appropriation and use of minerals (co-factors), you'll find that some of the benefits associated with certain vitamins may also be similar to some minerals).

As with minerals, there are two types of vitamins we need to be concerned with...

The first group are the fat-soluble vitamins, and these include Vitamins A, D, E and K. Fat-soluble vitamins can be stored by the body in reasonable amounts.

The other type we need are water-soluble vitamins, and these include Vitamin C and the B group vitamins. With the exception of Vitamin B12, the body cannot store any of these vitamins. [3,23]

Both types are still needed, however, and as I've already said a deficiency of any of the essential vitamins can, and eventually will, have a serious detrimental effect on one's overall health, well-being and longevity potential.

So here they are in no particular order...

Vitamin A (Retinol):

This vitamin is imperative for overall good health, youthfulness, and for increasing our life expectancy. It helps the body build a strong resistance to all types of infections, as well as protecting us against the harmful effects of pollution.

Vitamin A plays a fundamental role in keeping the epithelial tissues throughout the body healthy (lining of the stomach, lungs, intestines, urinary tract, vagina, bladder, eyes and skin). As a vast majority of cancers that occur in humans are malignancies of the epithelial tissues, it's therefore considered an *essential* nutrient for cancer prevention.

Retinol also plays an important role in normal teeth and bone development, along with helping the body maintain healthy reproductive organs. [3,23]

Vitamin A has a particular duty to perform in the retina of the eye – hence the name "retinol." It prevents eye diseases such as cataracts, as well as treating night blindness, poor eyesight and eye inflammation. A prolonged lack of vitamin A can lead to blindness. [3,23]

Beta-Carotene for Vitamin A

Vitamin A is one nutrient that can be toxic to the body in excessively high doses. The safest way to obtain this vitamin is from the carotenoid known as beta-carotene. The body is able to easily convert beta-carotene to vitamin A and safely excrete any excess.

You may have been told that eating carrots is good for your eyesight. Carrots are incredibly rich in beta-carotene (and therefore vitamin A).

But that's not all beta-carotene is good for...

A 19-year University study showed that beta-carotene dramatically reduces the risk of lung cancer, even in cigarette smokers. And the National Cancer Institute in Maryland, USA, also recently reported that consuming a diet high in beta-carotene can reduce one's risk of developing certain types of cancers by more than 40%! (Good thing wheat grass and barley grass contain more than *twice* the amount of beta-carotene than regular carrots). [3]

Other ailments and problems caused by a vitamin A deficiency include: retarded growth in children, bronchial complaints, frequent colds and flu, certain skin disorders, rough dry skin, and acne. [3,23]

Vitamin C:

Vitamin C is vitally important for the healthy functioning of *all* body cells. It assists the body in fighting infection and disease, mainly due to the strong effect it has on the action of the white blood cells.

Vitamin C helps with the synthesis of various hormones including the regulation of adrenal hormone production, along with being one of the essential components of collagen - the protein that gives us healthy skin, bones, cartilage, teeth and gums. It also helps maintain the elasticity of the skin, along with the arteries and tendons, and assists in the healing of all types of wounds and burns. [3,23]

Vitamin C is another nutrient that has been found to reduce blood cholesterol levels and improve glucose intolerance in diabetics. New studies have shown that it may help reduce the risk of cancer of the gastrointestinal tract by preventing dietary nitrates from turning into dangerous cancer-causing "nitrosamines." [3,23]

Vitamin C for a Strong Immune System...

Vitamin C is one of the most effective antioxidants available and plays an important role in protecting the body from the damaging effects of toxic chemicals contained in our food, water and air. It boosts the immune system tremendously and has a unique ability to reduce the duration and severity of the common cold and flu viruses. In fact, it's one of the most important anti-viral nutrients discovered thus far (together with zinc)!

Also known as an "anti-stress" nutrient, Vitamin C helps protect the body from all types of physical and mental stress, along with helping promote sound sleep. After studying this nutrient for many years, twice Nobel Prize winner, Professor Linus Pauling, published various books and clinical papers confirming the absolute necessity of vitamin C for overall good health and longevity. [3,23]

Other ailments and problems caused by a vitamin C deficiency include: fatigue, cataracts, glaucoma, and scurvy. [3,23]

Vitamin D:

As important as all of the essential vitamins are, if you had to pick **the** most important and crucial vitamin for perfect health, vitamin D would surely be it!

The number of illnesses and diseases this nutrient can help prevent and treat is astounding. Vitamin D is currently the hottest and most talked about topic in the alternative health industry with over 3000 scientific papers produced last year alone on its health and healing benefits. The main papers presented so far have been for cancer prevention and treatment, but there's plenty of others.

Here's just a few…

Alzheimer's and Dementia:

A 2014 study published in the *Neurology* journal found that a vitamin D deficiency in older adults can **double** the risk of some forms of dementia, including Alzheimer's disease. According to the study, people who have low levels of vitamin D are 70% more likely to develop Alzheimer's disease - and incredibly, those who are severely deficient are 120% more likely to develop Alzheimer's disease! [47]

Heart Disease:

According to research presented at the American College of Cardiology's Annual Scientific Session, a lack of vitamin D has been linked to cases of acute heart disease. Researchers found that over 70% of heart attack patients who underwent a coronary angiography (imaging used to see how blood is flowing through the arteries) had a chronic vitamin D deficiency. [47]

Schizophrenia:

A study published in the *Journal of Clinical Endocrinology & Metabolism* found that people who are vitamin D deficient are **twice** as likely to be diagnosed with schizophrenia compared to those with adequate levels. Researchers reviewed findings from 19 observational studies that looked at the relationship between schizophrenia and vitamin D to come to these results. [47]

Erectile Dysfunction:

A recent study published in the *Journal of Sexual Medicine* revealed that men with severe erectile dysfunction (ED) have significantly lower levels of vitamin D than men with only mild ED. Researchers said…

"Our study shows that a significant proportion of ED patients have a vitamin D deficiency and that this condition is more frequent in patients with the arteriogenic etiology (the main type of impotence which results when the arteries to the penis do not supply enough blood to cause an erection). Low levels of vitamin D might increase the ED risk by promoting endothelial dysfunction. Men with ED should be analyzed for vitamin D levels and particularly to A-ED patients with a low level a vitamin D supplementation is suggested". [47]

Osteoporosis and Arthritis:

Both of these diseases have been "overwhelmingly" proven to be caused by a calcium, magnesium, boron and vitamin D deficiency. Most people are already aware that vitamin D is essential for healthy bones, but not many are aware they can actually treat these diseases successfully by simply supplementing with 5000 IU's (international units) of vitamin D3 per day.

Premature Births:

Two researchers, Carol Wagner and Bruce Hollis, studied the effects of vitamin D on pregnant women. What they discovered was impressive. By simply giving 4,000 IU's of vitamin D daily to a group of pregnant women, they were able to lower their rate of preterm deliveries by an incredible 50%. Vitamin D has also been found to significantly lower a woman's chance of delivering a low weight baby, as well as reducing their risk of requiring a C-section during labor. [48]

Cancer:

Vitamin D has been found to be particularly effective for preventing and treating cancer, especially pancreatic, colon, lung, ovarian, skin, breast and prostate cancers. As a matter of fact, one study showed that women can lower their rate of **all** cancers, most notably breast cancer, by an astonishing 77%, simply by supplementing with vitamin D3 every day. And a male study, published in the *Journal of Clinical Oncology*, found that men with optimum levels of vitamin D in their blood were **half** as likely to get prostate cancer as men with low levels. [49]

It's interesting to note here that so far experts have identified 17 varieties of human cancers that can be prevented and even treated with regular sun exposure (for vitamin D production) along with taking vitamin D3 supplements. [49]

Other diseases and ailments caused by a vitamin D deficiency include: diabetes, rickets, high blood pressure, obesity, metabolic syndrome, multiple sclerosis, bursitis, gout, infertility, PMS, Parkinson's disease, depression, chronic fatigue syndrome, fibromyalgia, periodontal disease, Crohn's disease, asthma, and allergies, along with auto-immune diseases such as psoriasis, eczema, rosacea and rheumatoid arthritis. [49]

Vitamin E:

This vitamin is probably the most well known and vital antioxidant there is alongside vitamin C and selenium. It plays a fundamental role in protecting our cells from free radical damage, along with preventing unwanted problems such as premature ageing and diseases like cancer and heart disease.

It's especially important for protecting the body's cell membranes, DNA, fats and enzymes from damage, and for this reason, is considered to be the number one antioxidant choice. [3,23]

Back in 1993, Harvard Medical School and the National Institutes of Health came out with an interesting article titled *"An Anti-Cancer Diet Has Been Found"*. This article stemmed from a huge study that involved 29,000 people from the Ki Non Province in China, where they have the highest rate of cancer in the world. In the study, researchers gave all participants three key nutrients; vitamin E, beta carotene and selenium. Nothing else was altered in their diet or environment.

The result? Deaths from *all* cancers immediately went down by 13%, which in the context and enormity of the study (and the amount of study participants involved) was massive! [14]

Vitamin E for Circulation...

Vitamin E is also known as an anti-coagulant nutrient and helps prevent death through clotting in the blood vessels (thrombosis). It's therefore considered essential for normal blood circulation and for the healthy maintenance of the heart and arteries. [25]

A recent study conducted by scientists at England's Cambridge University confirms this:

The study, which involved 2,002 patients with various heart conditions, was able to overwhelmingly prove the value of vitamin E in helping patients with heart problems.

One of the researchers, Professor Morris Brown, commented after the study that he and his colleagues were "very excited" to discover that vitamin E really is as beneficial as they had hoped. He also said that he would be recommending vitamin E to angina patients as well as those at risk of heart disease. [25]

And in the Cambridge Heart and Antioxidant study, Dr Steven Nigel, who studied over 2000 patients with known coronary heart disease, gave one part of his group 400 IU's (international units) of vitamin E and the other group a placebo.

After following them for 18 months, he found the vitamin E group had 77% fewer heart attacks than the placebo group! [21]

Vitamin E Protects the Lungs

Further research carried out on vitamin E has showed it to be beneficial in the treatment of emphysema and protecting lung tissue from damage as a result of breathing in polluted air. Other studies have shown that vitamin E may help reduce the incidence of breast cancer in women, along with reducing the number and size of breast cysts.

Vitamin E is also essential for the healthy maintenance of our skin, liver, eyes and muscles. It's known to help increase sperm count in men as well as assist women with infertility problems. [3,23]

Vitamin E for Alzheimer's Disease...

Amazingly, sixty years ago in the animal industry farmers were able to prevent, treat and even cure Alzheimer's disease in animals by feeding them high doses of vitamin E.

As a result of recent studies carried out on human patients (we're obviously a little slower to catch up) this nutrient has now become recognized as a prevention and viable treatment for Alzheimer's disease in humans. [1]

In fact, after a recent study on Alzheimer's disease and vitamin E the University of California and the Salk Institute actually came out and said: *"Vitamin E eases memory loss in Alzheimer's patients."* And back in November of 2003, a further study was able to confirm that just by taking some supplemental vitamin E, you're 78% less likely to get Alzheimer's disease! [19,26,27]

Other problems caused by a vitamin E deficiency include: varicose veins, fatigue, asthma, miscarriages, and stillbirths. [3,23]

Vitamin B1 (Thiamine):

One of thiamine's main functions is to help the body convert carbohydrates and fats into energy, making it an important nutrient for increasing stamina and delaying the onset of fatigue. It also helps to prevent the toxic build up of by-products that accumulate from metabolism, therefore protecting the heart muscle and nervous system from systemic damage. [3,23]

Thiamine is known to stimulate the action of the brain as well as assist the body with normal growth and development. It helps promote better circulation and is beneficial for the prevention and treatment of certain heart conditions and digestive disorders. This essential nutrient is largely responsible for us maintaining our zest and youthful vitality. [3,23]

Other ailments and problems caused by a thiamine deficiency include: poor memory, constipation, irritability, mental depression, nervous exhaustion, and loss of appetite. [3,23]

Vitamin B2 (Riboflavin):

As with thiamine, riboflavin is also a vital component of energy metabolism. It plays a key role in the releasing of energy from food and regulation of thyroid activity, thus exerting a powerful and positive influence on stamina, vitality and mental acuteness. [3,23]

Riboflavin is extremely important for the health of the eyes and is known to help with preventing and even treating certain eye disorders, including cataracts. It also acts as an antioxidant and is necessary for maintaining a healthy immune system, normal growth and development, and for overall good health. [3,23]

Other problems and ailments caused by a riboflavin deficiency include: bloodshot eyes, abnormal sensitivity to light, eczema (itchy and inflamed skin), vaginal itching, ulcers, and premature wrinkles. [3,23]

Vitamin B3 (Niacin):

Niacin is a co-enzyme that's involved in the manufacturing of energy from carbohydrates, proteins and fats.

It's needed by the body to form neurotransmitters, making it crucial for the healthy functioning of the brain and nervous system. For this reason, B3 has been found to be helpful in the treatment of certain neurological problems such as nervousness, irritability, forgetfulness, depression, insomnia and mental disease. [3,23]

Niacin is also crucial for normal blood circulation and for maintaining a healthy digestive system. It aids in the health and upkeep of the skin, hair and eyes and is known to be useful in the treatment of mouth ulcers and for relieving cold hands and feet. [3,23]

Other ailments and problems caused by a niacin deficiency include: fatigue, constipation, skin rash, and migraine headaches.

Vitamin B5 (Pantothenic Acid):

This vitamin also forms part of the co-enzymes that are needed by the body to release energy from food.

It helps activate the adrenal glands (which are important for producing cortisone and other necessary hormones) and is a valuable nutrient in the fight against premature ageing, particularly the development of skin wrinkles and crow's feet around the eyes. [3,23]

Studies have shown that pantothenic acid can help ward off bodily infections *and* speed up the recovery rate from illness. It's imperative for the healthy development of the entire nervous system and plays a fundamental role in protecting the body against most forms of physical and mental stress. [3,23]

Other problems and ailments caused by a B5 deficiency include: chronic fatigue, allergies, asthma, mental depression, insomnia, irritability, constipation, skin disorders, hypoglycemia (low blood sugar), low blood pressure, and retarded growth. [3,23]

Vitamin B6 (Pyridoxine):

Pyridoxine is important for the manufacturing of antibodies, which guard against harmful bacterial invasions. B6, along with niacin, is needed for the formation of neurotransmitters, making it essential for the health and correct functioning of the nervous system and brain. Recent studies have shown that pyridoxine not only assists with many nervous disorders, it may help lessen and even prevent some forms of epileptic seizures. [3,23]

Another major benefit of B6 lies in its ability to protect the body against certain types of degenerative diseases and ailments including arteriosclerosis, heart disorders, elevated cholesterol levels and diabetes. It's also known to help with overweight problems caused by edema (fluid retention) along with helping prevent pre-menstrual edema. [3,23]

Pyridoxine is important for healthy pregnancies, protecting teeth against tooth decay and in the prevention and treatment of kidney stones. It's a crucial nutrient for protein and fat metabolism (especially essential fatty acids) and for the production and synthesis of DNA and RNA. [3,23]

Other ailments caused by a pyridoxine deficiency include: anemia, mental depression, insomnia, nervousness, cramps, and skin disorders such as acne. [3,23]

Vitamin B12 (Cyanocobalamin):

Vitamin B12 is required for the normal development and workings of all body cells. It plays a significant role in the manufacture and regeneration of red blood cells and a deficiency is known to cause pernicious anaemia. B12 is also necessary for maintaining the health of the tissues of the bones, nerves, reproductive organs and gastrointestinal tract. [3,23]

Vitamin B12 works in combination with the other B group vitamins in helping to release energy from food. It's vital for the production of myelin (the white sheath that surrounds nerve fibres) and a deficiency can result in damage to the nervous system, along with causing chronic fatigue (CFS) and loss of mental acuity. [3,23]

(*Note*: Recent laboratory analysis have shown that although plant foods are usually devoid of vitamin B12, dehydrated wheat grass and barley grass actually contain high amounts of B12. Fermented lactobacillus foods are also a rich source of this important nutrient.)

Other problems caused by a B12 deficiency include: numbness or stiffness, concentration difficulties, poor appetite, and slow growth in children. [3,23]

Folate (Folic Acid):

Folic acid is one nutrient that is certainly lacking from our modern day diets. It works together with B12 to form red blood cells and a deficiency results in a type of anemia where the red blood cells become abnormally large and incorrectly formed (macrocytic anemia).

Without folic acid our bodies are unable to produce enough antibodies to fight off infection. This makes it essential for the health of the immune system, and in fact, our body's entire growth and healing process. [3,23]

Folate for Healthy Pregnancies...

Folate is definitely one of the most important and critical nutrients for reproductive health and healthy pregnancies.

Studies have now been able to prove that a daily intake of folic acid can greatly reduce the risk of women bearing a child with spina bifida or other neural tube defects by as much as 90%!

In addition, there is now substantial evidence showing that folate can help prevent foetal malformations and spontaneous abortions during pregnancies. A deficiency can also result in a long and difficult labour and has been linked to high infant death rates. [3,18,23]

Other problems caused by a folate deficiency include: skin disorders, greying hair, poor circulation, stomach irritation, and fatigue. [3,23]

Biotin:

This nutrient is vital for the healthy maintenance of the skin, hair and nails. Combined with the trace mineral tin, it's instrumental in preventing excessive hair loss and slowing down the signs of male pattern baldness.

Studies have indicated that hair loss may actually result from a by-product of the hormone testosterone. This by-product causes a shrivelling of the hair follicle and prevents new hair growth. Biotin is able to neutralize this substance, and in turn, allow the hair to continue to grow and remain healthy. [3,23]

Biotin is also needed for the metabolic process that releases energy from proteins, carbohydrates and fats. It's important for the heart and lungs and a deficiency can lead to various skin problems including dermatitis, eczema and dandruff, along with other skin disorders such as pallor. [3,23]

Other problems caused by a biotin deficiency include: anaemia, mental depression, conjunctivitis, muscle pain, and loss of appetite. [3,23]

Vitamin K:

Vitamin K is an essential nutrient for blood clotting.

One important and somewhat miraculous function of the blood lies in its ability to clot when required, which of course prevents dangerous health problems such as hemorrhaging and excessive blood loss from occurring. This process, however, *cannot* be performed correctly without adequate levels of Vitamin K in the blood!

Vitamin K is routinely given to newborn babies to prevent a potentially life-threatening hemorrhagic disease that can sometimes occur during the first few weeks of life. It's also of particular benefit to the millions of women who suffer monthly with menstrual problems such as excessive menstrual flow and menstrual cramps. [23,28]

Apart from blood clotting, Vitamin K is needed for bone metabolism and proper kidney function. A deficiency can result in many blood associated problems such as excessive bruising, spontaneous bleeding and excessive bleeding from slight injuries (many of which are routinely seen in the elderly).

In addition to these, a vitamin K deficiency can accompany ailments such as cystic fibrosis, prolonged diarrhea and liver disease. Vitamin K2 is also essential for the correct absorption and utilization of vitamin D in the blood (thankfully, both wheat grass and barley grass are rich sources of this critical nutrient as well!). [23,28]

Choline:

The major role of choline is to control fat transportation and metabolism in the body. It helps prevent fat and cholesterol from forming in the liver and blood stream - so this nutrient is of immense benefit to anyone suffering from high cholesterol, "fatty liver" disease, or other health problems caused by excessive fat intake. (Of course, if you did suffer from any of these ailments then your first course of action would be to cut out all bad fats from your diet). [3]

Choline is also an important nutrient for the nerves and is needed for the maintenance and growth of nerve tissue and regulation of nerve transmission. It's been found to be beneficial in the treatment of many different disorders including gallstones, glaucoma, liver disorders, hardening of the arteries and kidney problems. [3]

Bioflavonoids:

The main purpose of bioflavonoids is to help with the absorption and utilisation of Vitamin C. In fact, these nutrients are able to fortify vitamin C's effect <u>a thousand fold</u> - substantially increasing its potency and beneficial properties.

Bioflavonoids help to strengthen the walls of the blood vessels and reduce capillary fragility. They act as anti-coagulants and are beneficial in the prevention and healing of arterial blood clots (coronary thrombosis) and strokes. [3]

Bioflavonoids are also known to aid in the prevention and treatment of other blood and circulatory problems including varicose veins, bleeding gums, hemorrhaging, hardening of the arteries, hemorrhoids, susceptibility to bruising, psoriasis and eczema.

Blood vessel disorders can play a major role in the development of other health problems such as retinal (eye) inflammation, hypertension, diabetes, premature aging, rheumatoid arthritis, miscarriage, bleeding ulcers and liver cirrhosis - so bioflavonoids may be of assistance in the prevention and management of these ailments as well. [3]

Other Vital Vitamins and Close Relatives:

Inositol is another vitamin known to help reduce high cholesterol levels and fat absorption in the blood.

P.A.B.A (Para-Amino-Benzoic Acid) is a strong anti-aging nutrient that helps prevent unwanted skin changes caused by aging along with reversing premature greying of the hair. [3]

Then there's the more recently discovered nutrients known as lycopenes (these compounds are actually carotenoids and technically not classed as vitamins, however, I've included them here as vitamins are the carotenoid's closest relatives). Along with vitamin D, these substances have also become the latest "talk" around the health and healing circles as they've been found to protect us from everything from heart disease, to skin and prostate cancer, along with a whole bunch of other deadly cancers! [19,27]

The List of Vitamins and Their Health and Healing Benefits Continues on...

Now, at the risk of sounding like a broken record, I'm only going to say this one more time... Making sure you receive *all* 16 vitamins every day from natural food sources such as wheat grass and a high quality lactobacillus rich food is absolutely crucial to your overall health, well-being and longevity potential!

In fact, I liken it to your body's need for oxygen.

We all know that without a sufficient supply of oxygen we would slowly suffocate and eventually die.

Well, without a sufficient supply of vitamins our bodies will also eventually suffocate and die before their time.

The only difference is that with a lack of vitamins our death will be a lot slower (and more painful) than what it would be with a lack of oxygen!

* * *

So now that we know the "why" and "how" of our need for vitamins and minerals every day, the next type of nutrients we need to be concerned with are amino acids.

Known as "the building blocks of life," amino acids have finally been recognized for the many healthy and positive benefits they exert on our bodies.

Let's discover why...

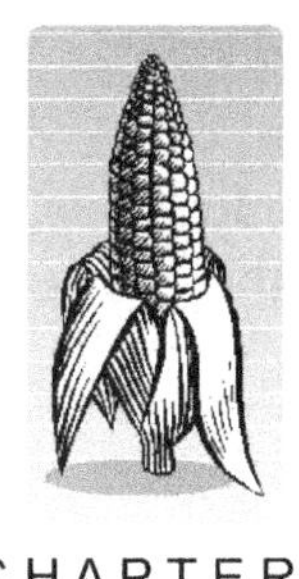

CHAPTER 6

Live Longer and Stronger With Key Macronutrients...

When it comes to macronutrients, you may have heard the word "amino acids" mentioned many times and know they relate to protein in some way, but do you know exactly *what* they are?

Amino acids are basically the "building blocks" or key components of protein.

After water, protein is the second most abundant substance in the body and actually makes up over half of the dry weight of human bodies.

Muscles, skin, hair, eyes, nails, and all of our internal organs, are mostly protein. Protein is the main substance that gives structure to virtually every living thing. [3,11]

The human body though requires thousands of *different* proteins in order to function correctly at any given time. It's a big demand, and because the body cannot immediately use proteins from outside sources (food), it has to *first* break them down into their key components (amino acids) and then recombine them to form the new proteins it needs. [3,11]

Obviously, if the body doesn't receive an adequate supply of protein, and subsequently, amino acids, then this whole process becomes greatly impaired and the end result can be chronic illness and disease.

Health Problems Caused From Amino Acid Deficiencies...

It's interesting to note that amino acid deficiencies have now become one of the *major* causes of some of the most common health problems we see in society today, some of which include; chronic fatigue, sleeping disorders, digestive problems, skin ailments, obesity, reduced energy levels, malnourishment, and a serious build up of wastes in the bloodstream. [3,11]

There are also many psychological problems that accompany amino acid deficiencies as well such as emotional upsets, depression, nervousness, and a general state of poor mental health.[3,11]

So the necessity of having a sufficient amount of protein (and therefore amino acids) in the diet is of utmost importance.

Remember this... the human body is continuously busy repairing and rebuilding itself, 24 hours a day, 7 days a week.

All of this rebuilding and repair work requires amino acids!

Also remember that without amino acids the correct assimilation and utilisation of other important nutrients, particularly vitamins and minerals, is severely impacted as well (for instance, methionine is needed for the absorption of zinc and selenium). [11]

Why We Need Amino Acids...

Amino acids are required for several basic and crucial functions in the body. Some of these include:

- The promotion of growth and healing of the cells and tissues;

- The formation of infection-fighting antibodies;

- Manufacturing of enzymes for digestion;

- The production of hormones - making them vital for reproduction;

- Formation of neurotransmitters;

- Contributing to the functions of the bloodstream;

- Preservation of electrolyte/water balance and acid/alkaline balance;

- Providing energy. [3,11,28]

There are about 20 different amino acids that make up proteins. The human body is able to make 80% of these, which are called non-essential. The remaining 20% must be obtained from the foods we consume and are known as essential amino acids.

Opinions concerning the actual number of essential amino acids the body requires each day varies, but it's somewhere within the range of 8 to 12. [11,28]

Not All Proteins Are The Same...

Now, nutritionists know that "all proteins are not created equal." The body is able to utilize proteins from some foods better than others.

It's also known that food proteins cannot be properly utilized by the body unless *all* essential amino acids are present in appropriate amounts. These types of proteins are called complete proteins. When a protein is deficient in one or more amino acids it's known as an incomplete protein.

Most animal proteins are known as complete proteins, whereas plant proteins are considered to be incomplete.

Wheat grass and barley grass are the exception though. They both contain *all* of the essential amino acids in proportions that make them very useable by the body (over 90% useable). And they boast good amounts of all the non-essential amino acids too! [28]

Specific Functions and Therapeutic Benefits of Amino Acids...

Research into the therapeutic use and benefits of amino acids during the past twenty to thirty years has been intense.

Much of this research has been carried out by Dr Eric Braverman from the Princeton Brain Bio Centre. [11]

The results have been so positive that there are now many practitioners using amino acid therapy on their patients to combat a wide range of health problems, rather than resorting to drug therapy.

The success rate has been outstanding, and as a result, we're beginning to see a gradual rise in the popularity of amino acid therapy - not just in America and Europe, but right around the world.

The word is finally getting out!

So let's have a look at some of the specific functions and therapeutic benefits of the most common essential and non-essential amino acids in more detail…

L-Arginine:

Arginine is one of the most well-known amino acids, particularly within the health and fitness industry. It helps with the detoxification and filtering of poisonous wastes and harmful substances out of the body. It's also important for normal growth and development, strong immune function and DNA synthesis.

Research has found that arginine is involved in the stimulation of the growth hormone somatotropin, which helps build lean muscle and burn body fat. For this reason, arginine supplementation is a favorite amongst bodybuilders and other strength athletes. [3,11]

Studies have shown that arginine can slow down and inhibit the growth of tumors and may even help with reducing the development of breast cancer cells. It has a positive effect on sperm production in adult males - so it helps prevent and even treat male infertility.

Arginine is also regularly prescribed by natural health practitioners for the treatment of erectile dysfunction. In a study published in the *Journal of Sex & Marital Therapy* back in 2003, Bulgarian researchers discovered that when arginine and pycnogenol (pine bark, grape seed extract) were given to erectile dysfunction sufferers, all participants reported a major improvement in sexual desire and sexual function, with no side effects. [54]

Low levels of arginine have also been associated with obesity, weight fluctuations, hypoglycemia, high blood pressure and high cholesterol. [3,11]

L-Alanine:

Alanine is an important nutrient for reducing cholesterol levels. Studies show that alanine, arginine and glycine combined can reduce cholesterol levels by 20-50% (all three amino acids are contained in wheat grass in generous amounts.) [28]

Alanine plays a crucial role in the regulation of blood-sugar levels, and as such, is beneficial in the treatment of diabetes and hyperactivity. Further research has shown it may be useful in the treatment of some forms of epilepsy, and because it contributes to thymus growth, can help patients with immune deficiencies.

Alanine is also found abundantly in muscle tissue and is an important amino acid for energy production. [3,11]

L-Cysteine:

Cysteine is a potent antioxidant. It combines with glutamic acid and glycine (two other amino's) to stimulate and build-up the body's immune system, which in turn gives strong protection against harmful bacterial and viral infections.

Cysteine is also imperative for ridding the body of ingested poisons from the gastrointestinal tract, as well as eliminating any foreign bacteria and toxins that may find their way into the bloodstream. It works with Vitamins B1 and C to protect the cells from the harmful effects of radiation and the toxic compounds found in cigarette smoke and polluted air. [3,11]

Because cysteine is able to bind to heavy metals such as arsenic, lead, mercury and cadmium (and drag them out of the body), their damaging effects are also greatly reduced.

L-Glutamine:

Known as "brain fuel," glutamine is one of only a small number of compounds capable of crossing the blood-brain barrier and participating in brain chemistry.

When it enters the brain, glutamine is converted into glutamic acid, where it then acts as an energy source for brain metabolism. It also absorbs ammonia - a toxic by-product of protein metabolism, which if left to accumulate, can severely damage the brain. [3,11]

Glutamine is *vital* for efficient brain functioning and "clear thinking." It's well known for its ability to raise a person's IQ and speed up and improve memory recall and learning abilities in both adults and children. [3,11]

Studies by Dr William Shive at the University of Texas have indicated that glutamine may be helpful in the healing of peptic ulcers. It's also been used successfully to curb alcohol cravings and is thought to help protect cells from the damage caused by excessive alcohol consumption. [3,11]

Other ailments that glutamine may assist with include: depression, mental fatigue and learning disabilities.

L-Histidine:

Histidine could technically be considered an essential amino acid, even though adults are able to make small amounts.

Studies have shown that histidine can repair tissue damage, making it a valuable nutrient in the treatment of rheumatoid arthritis along with conditions such as anemia and seasonal allergies.

Histidine has also been found to be beneficial in the treatment of prostate gland problems including prostatitis (swollen prostate). [3,11]

L-Isoleucine/L-Leucine/L-Valine:

These three essential amino acids are known as branched-chain amino's or BCAA's.

Structurally, BCAA's are very similar to each other but are

metabolised in a different way to other amino acids. The body's requirement for branched-chain amino's is also higher, particularly during states of intense stress and before and after physical exercise. They're all needed for protein synthesis, the re-utilization of amino acids and for minimising protein breakdown. [3,11]

Diseases that have been treated successfully with these amino acids include hepatitis, liver disease and cirrhosis. Valine in particular has been found to be highly beneficial in the treatment of an ailing liver. Research has shown that people with Parkinson's disease and eating disorders also have low levels of these three amino acids. [3,11]

Isoleucine is important for the formation of hemoglobin in the blood, regulating blood sugar and energy levels, and for maintaining sound mental health.

Leucine is needed for the maintenance of tissue health and the lowering of blood sugar levels if they become too high.

Valine acts as a natural stimulant and is vital for the successful functioning of the nervous system. It's required for tissue regeneration, along with maintaining positive nitrogen balance (PNB results in increased muscle development and better coordination). Valine is also directly associated with maintaining strong mental vigor and a deficiency is characterized by neurological defects in the brain. [3,11]

L-Lysine:

Lysine is an essential nutrient needed by the body for growth, tissue repair and the production of antibodies to fight illness and disease. It's been well documented for its ability to control viral infections including the herpes simplex virus, canker sores and cold sores.

Lysine is also important for healthy reproduction, normal functioning of the nervous system and red blood cell production. Recent studies have shown that lysine may even help prevent tooth decay. [3,11]

L-Methionine:

An essential amino acid, methionine is an exceptionally powerful detoxification agent. It plays a fundamental role in protecting and removing poisons from the liver as well as actually promoting cell regeneration of the liver and kidneys.

Methionine helps break down fats in the body and is involved in allowing the liver to burn fat at an increased rate. This amino acid has also been found to help alleviate arthritic-rheumatic disorders in the elderly. [3,11]

L-Phenylalanine:

Phenylalanine is another amino acid that is extremely beneficial and "highly stimulating" to the central nervous system of the brain. Known to help "pick you up" it increases mental alertness and significantly improves learning and memory functions.

Phenylalanine also acts as a strong pain reliever and anti-depressant. Studies show that it offers sustained relief from chronic pain including lower back pain, arthritis, and migraine headaches - due in part to its ability to inhibit the enzymes that normally break down enkephalins – the body's natural morphine-like pain killers. Other research conducted showed phenylalanine to be *over 80%* effective in cases of depression! [3,11]

A further benefit of phenylalanine lies in its ability to release a hormone called CCK. This hormone acts as an appetite suppressant, so it naturally reduces the body's desire to consume large amounts of food. For people seeking to lose weight and trim down, this nutrient is a boon. [3,11]

NOTE: The phenylalanine contained in diet drinks and diet sodas is *not* healthy. Because it's been chemically altered, this form of phenylalanine is extremely toxic to the body and should be avoided completely!

L-Tyrosine:

Tyrosine, along with phenylalanine, has now become a proven alternative for helping control anxiety and depression rather than harmful anti-depressant drugs. Clinical studies have confirmed tyrosine's value in overcoming the symptoms of depression, particularly in regards to the use of oral contraceptives and the effects these medications can have on one's mood. [3,11]

Back in the 1980's, a ground-breaking article was published in the *American Journal of Psychiatry* by Dr Alan Gelenberg from Harvard Medical School. In the article, Dr Gelenberg was discussing the success he had with tyrosine in treating patients with long-term depression...

In short, he took patients who were not responding to depression medication and administered them with dietary supplements of tyrosine. Within a few weeks many patients were either able to reduce their intake of amphetamines to minimal levels or discontinue with the drugs altogether. [3,11]

Along with a reduction in depression and anxiety, an improvement in mental alertness and memory retainability has also been found with the supplemental use of tyrosine. It's known to help increase a person's overall mental attitude, as well as assist in the treatment of Parkinson's disease, high blood pressure and seasonal allergies. [3,11]

L-Tryptophan:

Tryptophan contributes to the production of the neurotransmitter hormone, serotonin, which is responsible for the regulation of moods, pain response and sleep.

Known as an "emotional stabilizer" tryptophan is renowned for its supreme calming effect, along with its ability to control depression and induce normal sleep patterns. After years of extensive research and testing in both Great Britain and the United States, tryptophan has *repeatedly* proven itself as a successful treatment for anxiety and sleeping disorders such as insomnia and sleep apnea. [3,11]

The beauty of tryptophan is it doesn't make you tired during the day, yet promotes restful sleep at night. And it has no harmful side effects, nor is it addictive and habit-forming like sleeping pills and other pharmaceutical relaxants.

When asked to comment on tryptophan therapy for combating emotional and sleeping problems, Dr Quentin Regestein from Harvard Medical School said: *"We have good grounds for hope that with L-tryptophan we will have a population which is free from hypnotics."* [3,11]

Tryptophan has also been used successfully in the treatment of other health disorders including anorexia nervosa, schizophrenia, respiratory disease, pancreatic disease and chronic pain. [3,11]

L-Taurine:

Even though taurine is not structurally part of the building blocks of protein, it's still an important amino acid.

Taurine is not only needed for maintaining the health of crucial organs such as the brain, heart, kidneys and gallbladder, it plays a *powerful* role in protecting and combating diseases in these organs as well.

Taurine is also known to act as an inhibitor for the excitatory functions of the nervous system and has proven to be enormously successful in the treatment of epileptic seizures, along with other nervous and muscular type disorders. [3,11]

Other ailments taurine is known to help with include: high blood pressure, gallstones, heart disease, arteriosclerosis, angina pectoris and mental fatigue.

NOTE: You'll find synthetic taurine added to many of the "energy drinks" on the market today. These horrible drinks fit into the same category as diet drinks (toxic and dangerous) and belong in the bin!

L-Threonine:

Threonine is an essential amino acid that's required for the digestive and intestinal tracts to function smoothly. It aids in the digestion of food and helps to improve the assimilation and absorption of valuable nutrients. Threonine also helps limit the amount of fat stored in the liver. [3,11]

The List Of Essential And Non-essential Amino Acids Goes On...

What's really exciting at the moment is because there's such a high degree of research being conducted on amino acids, and this research is finally confirming the therapeutic value of these essential nutrients, many in the medical field are literally being *forced* to stand up and take notice!

Since amino acid balances and imbalances can have such a

profound effect on illness and wellness within the human body, it's extremely critical that we receive a daily supply from whole foods such as wheat grass and barley grass - which is a nutritional resource of quality protein that many experts agree has barely been tapped!

Other good food sources of quality protein will be discussed more in Chapter 9.

* * *

So now that we know why our bodies need amino acids, and more importantly, what will happen if we don't receive a sufficient supply, the next type of nutrients we need everyday are essential fatty acids.

Just remember, not *all* fats are bad for you. As you'll soon discover, some fats actually have a very important role to play in our health and longevity.

Let's continue on to see why...

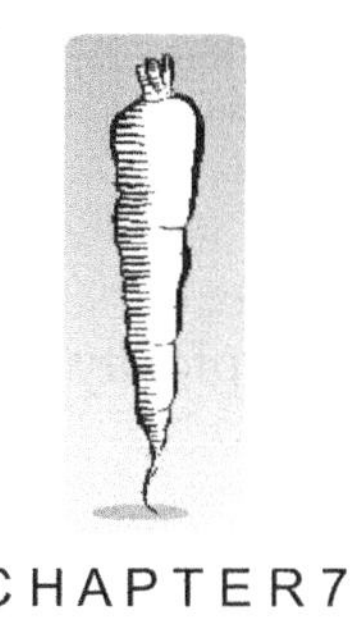

CHAPTER 7

Starve Off Alzheimer's, Dementia and Other Deadly Diseases With These Stunning Nutrients

The word "fat" has become a bit of a "dirty word" in society today. Even the mere mention of it can make many people cringe! That's because most people believe fat is bad for you and should be kept out of your diet.

This presumption is totally false.

The truth is there are "good fats" and "bad fats" and the beneficial ones, as their name suggests, are *essential* for the health and correct functioning of *all* body cells. In fact, a long-term deficiency of essential fatty acids can actually result in death! [29,30]

New research has found that these good fats have many positive benefits such as helping to prevent disease and accelerating the rate at which the body is able to burn fat (yes that's right, consuming fat to lose fat!). [29,30]

The Two Main Types of Fats...

There are two main types of fats we need to be concerned with;

saturated and unsaturated.

Saturated fats: These are typically classed as the bad ones, although not all of them *are* bad.

Basically, these types of fats contain the maximum amount of hydrogen atoms possible ("saturated" with hydrogen atoms), making them solid at room temperature.

A diet high in certain saturated fats, particularly those found in margarine, processed meats, and fried foods, can cause these fats to clump together and form deposits that lodge in the organs and blood vessels of the body. This can lead to many serious health problems including heart disease, "fatty liver," obesity, breast cancer, insulin resistance and colon cancer. [29,30]

Saturated fats found in foods such as coconut oil, peanut butter and avocados, however, can actually be beneficial.

In the *Journal of the American Medical Association* (J.A.M.A.) - one of the worlds most renowned medical journals - they released an article back in the late 1990's saying that if you *increase* your saturated fat intake from healthy food sources by 9% above the daily average, you can *decrease* your chance of stroke by 45%! [19]

And in a 2017 randomised trial, where they tested the implications of consuming coconut oil, olive oil (which also contains saturated fat) and butter, researchers found that butter increased LDL (bad cholesterol) levels slightly, olive oil made no difference, and surprisingly, coconut oil lowered LDL levels and raised HDL (good cholesterol) levels. [47]

It's also interesting to note that during the 1970's and early 80's, the peoples of Sri Lanka were the biggest consumers of coconut oil in the world, and coincidently, had the lowest rate of heart disease of any nation in the world. Sadly today, coconut oil is all but gone from their diets and they now consume harmful imported commercially processed oils (see below) like we do. Heart disease has now taken over as their number one killer. [48]

Unsaturated Fats: Unlike saturated fats, unsaturated fats do not contain the maximum amount of hydrogen atoms possible ("unsaturated" with hydrogen atoms) and are usually soft or liquid at room temperature.

These fats mainly come from sources such as vegetables and fish. Unsaturated fats are also subdivided into two categories – monounsaturated and polyunsaturated.

The body does not strictly need monounsaturated fats as it's able to manufacture them from carbohydrates and proteins. However, the body is unable to manufacture certain polyunsaturated fats (essential fatty acids) so these *must* come from the diet. [23]

The problem is the balance of fat intake in most people's diets today is tipped excessively high towards the "bad" saturated fats and tipped very low towards healthy fats (essential fatty acids).

Why Our Bodies Must Have Essential Fatty Acids (EFAs)

Essential fatty acids, like vitamins, minerals and amino acids, are important nutritional substances that are required for many bodily processes.

Research has shown that EFAs help with all of the following:

• Normal brain functioning;

• Correct hormone production;

• Reducing blood pressure;

• Lowering of cholesterol and triglyceride levels;

• Prostaglandin production;

• Maintaining healthy skin;

• Preventing and relieving arthritis, lupus, IBS and other inflammation-related ailments;

• Reducing the growth rate of breast cancer cells;

• Helping with transmission of nerve impulses;

• Helping with the construction of body membranes;

• Removing plaque from arterial walls;

• Mood regulation and enhancement. [30]

A deficiency of essential fatty acids is extremely common in industrialized countries like the United States, Great Britain, Australia, and many European nations. Factors such as stress, disease, allergies, and a diet high in processed foods, all increase the bodies need for essential fatty acids.

Because EFAs have so many functions to perform, there are many symptoms of essential fatty acid deficiencies, some of which include:

• Poor growth;

• Enlarged, fatty liver;

• Kidney problems;

• Skin disorders such as eczema, acne and psoriasis;

• Heart problems;

• Decreased capillary resistance;

• Anemia;

• Gallbladder dysfunction;

• Slow wound healing;

• Male and female infertility;

• Increased susceptibility to disease;

• Prostate inflammation;

• Cardiovascular disorders;

• Proneness to infection. [30]

The EFA Family...

There are two essential fatty acids the body requires everyday – omega-6 (linoleic acid or LA is the most common) and omega-3 - which includes alpha-linolenic acid (ALA), eicosapentaenoic acid (EPA) and docosahexaenoic acid (DHA).

Here's the main benefits of both...

Omega-6:

Linoleic acid is probably the most vital omega-6. LA is needed by the body to make two other important omega-6 fatty acids – arachidonic acid and gamma-linolenic acid (GLA). These two EFAs are particularly crucial to our health and well-being as they help the body maintain correct levels of important chemical substances known as prostaglandins. These hormone-like substances, which are manufactured purely from essential fatty acids, are needed to regulate every tissue and organ at the cellular level.

The benefits of prostaglandins are many: They help us sustain adequate energy levels by stimulating thyroid hormone production, along with blocking the body's overproduction of histamine – the chemical responsible for exacerbating allergic symptoms such as itchy and runny eyes, stuffy nose and scratchy throat.

Research has also found that low levels of prostaglandins may induce certain types of asthma. It was discovered when prostaglandin levels are maintained normal the muscles in the lungs are able to relax and blood flow is increased. [29,30]

One type of prostaglandin in particular, PGE1, has been noted for its vast array of health benefits. It does all of the following:

- Lowers blood pressure;

- Slows cholesterol production;

- Opens blood vessels;

- Relieves angina pain;

- Prevents inflammation;

- Controls arthritis;

- Enhances the effectiveness of insulin;

- Stops the growth of certain types of cancer cells;

- Strengthens the immune system;

- Produces a heightened sense of well-being. [29,30]

Because prostaglandins affect the body in so many ways, the importance of maintaining sufficient levels cannot be over emphasised. In fact, we open ourselves up to a large number of health problems if correct levels are *not* sustained.

It's also interesting to note that synthetic prostaglandin drugs have now been created for use in medicine. Using them does involve some risk, however, and they can have many undesirable effects on other bodily processes. It's therefore *much* safer to take a natural substance like evening primrose oil, which contains the EFAs needed by the body to produce prostaglandins naturally. [29,30]

Omega-3:

Alpha-linolenic acid is considered the most important of the omega-3's. The body uses ALA to make two other EFAs in the omega-3 family, eicosapentaenoic acid (EPA) and docosahexaenoic acid (DHA). These particular essential fatty acids are crucial for blood thinning and preventing abnormal blood clotting (thrombosis). ALA, EPA and DHA are all important for the regulation of cholesterol as they not only help *with* the production of cholesterol, but also the *removal* of excess cholesterol from the blood. [29]

Omega-3's strengthen the walls of the cells, providing protection from harmful viral and bacterial invasions. They naturally reduce inflammation and help tremendously in the treatment (and prevention) of heart disease, stroke, psoriasis and arthritis.

Many patients have in fact reported amazing relief from arthritis and psoriasis through the daily supplementation of omega-3's. And to top it off, a study back in November of 2003 found that supplementing with omega-3's can actually reduce your chance of getting Alzheimer's by a whopping 48%! [19,27]

The "Bad Fats" And Why We Must Avoid Them...

You don't need to be a rocket scientist to realize that bad fats are called "bad fats" for a reason. These types of fats include certain saturated fats, along with damaged fats that come from margarine, hydrogenated oils and commercially processed oils (which includes all fried foods).

There's now overwhelming evidence to prove that consuming these bad fats on a regular basis increases your chance of developing deadly diseases such as heart disease and cancer (by a significant amount). [23,29,30]

I've already spoken about good and bad saturated fats, but many people aren't aware of the dangers of hydrogenated oils, commercially processed oils and fried foods, so let's take a look at these in more detail...

What Are Hydrogenated Oils?

"Hydrogenation" is the method used to turn natural oils into the types of fats used in margarines and shortenings, along with most convenience foods such as biscuits, cakes, pies and packet chips. As a matter of fact, virtually *all* of the processed foods on the market today that contain fat contain hydrogenated oils!

The hydrogenation process was developed to enhance cooking appeal and lengthen shelf life. Unfortunately, hydrogenation also creates free radicals and trans-fatty acids. These substances are incredibly destructive and noxious to the body (due to the radical and unnatural chemical changes they undergo during processing).

Trans-fats are considered "foreign" by the body and create mass confusion for the cells - they simply don't know what to do with them. Often referred to as "plastic fats" (because they act like plastic in the body), trans-fatty acids create unhealthy cellular activity, interfere with prostaglandin production and make our blood platelets sticky, resulting in poor blood flow and increased blood clots. Trans-fats also lower your immunity, liver function, fat metabolism and body energy production. [23,29,30]

Trans-fatty acids have been in the spotlight for some time (for all the wrong reasons) and are regarded as one of the prime suspects in the development of heart disease. The results of a large study published in *The New England Journal of Medicine* showed that regular consumption of trans-fatty acids causes cholesterol and LDL fat levels in the blood to rise to exceedingly high levels. Of course, these factors are known to greatly increase one's risk of developing cardiovascular disease. [23,29,30]

And in the famous *Harvard Medical Nurses' Health Study* - where 121,000 nurses were studied for 20 years - they found the participants who regularly consumed the "king" of trans-fatty oils, margarine, had 75% **more** cardiovascular disease and heart disease than those who consumed butter! [19,27]

So What's Wrong With Commercially Processed Oils Then?

One very important and crucial factor about oils containing EFAs is they are only beneficial when consumed in their *natural state.*

Essential fatty acids deteriorate rapidly when exposed to air, light and heat. The extraction and refining methods that are used for commercially processed oils subjects them to all three!

All that matters with mass market refining is getting the job done quickly and cheaply. Retaining the health qualities of the oils are not considered nor cared about.

Commercially processed oils are manufactured under extremely high temperatures, which destroy the nutritional qualities of EFAs and create toxic trans-fatty acids.

The breaking down process and oxidation of the oil causes dangerous chemicals such as polymers, hydroperoxyaldehydes and peroxides to form. The oil can also contain chemical residues as a result of the petroleum (petrochemical) solvents that are used during the extraction process.

Even when the processing is over, further damage continues to occur. The oil is exposed to light through the bottles (these bottles should be dark to block out light), which results in the production of cancer-causing free radicals and pro-oxidants.

The bottles then sit on the shelf of the supermarket, becoming exposed to more light - and once opened, further oxidation of the oil begins to take place. [29,30]

Finally, when the oil is heated and used for cooking, it increases the production of harmful trans-fatty acids *A THOUSAND FOLD!* [19,27]

This is why fried foods (especially deep-fried foods) pose such a serious danger to our health.

Commercially processed oils are used in the cooking of fried foods. And in most commercial restaurants and fast-food places, these oils are *repeatedly* re-used and heated to high temperatures. Not only does this result in dangerous levels of trans- fats, but other deadly chemicals such as cyclic monomers and heterocyclic amines also accumulate in the oil. [19,27]

Fried foods, especially deep-fried foods, *should not be eaten*, and if you have liver or gallbladder problems, *do not* eat fried foods ever!

Replacing Your Fats and Oils...

Commercially processed oils that come from canola, corn, soy, cottonseed, rice bran, sunflower and safflower are all <u>extremely</u> carcinogenic and should be thrown away and replaced with unrefined cold pressed oils in dark bottles (you can usually find these in the health food isle of your supermarket). These oils can then be used on salad dressings, added to homemade cakes, and used for light stir-frying.

Cooking can be done by using no oil at all or using coconut oil (coconut oil can be safely heated to high temperatures). If you must use a vegetable oil, use virgin olive oil and stir fry your food like the Chinese do. They use water and oil together, constantly stirring the food while cooking. This keeps the temperature of the oil lower and prevents the oxidation and production of trans-fatty acids. [30]

Hydrogenated vegetable oils, margarines and shortenings are the last type of bad fats that need to be kept to a zero level.

A good practice is to read labels on processed foods (if you must eat them) so you know what hydrogenated oils, vegetable oils, etc, are in them.

I do understand that we're all human though and trying to eat a perfect diet and avoid the unhealthy fats all of the time is virtually impossible.

Thankfully, the daily consumption of essential fatty acids can help offset much of the damage that can be done by the bad fats.

Where to Obtain Your Essential Fatty Acids From...

The ratio in which our bodies need EFAs is roughly 3:1 – meaning, we should be consuming around three omega-6 to one omega-3. Unfortunately, the current ratio for the standard Westernized diet is around 16:1, which is way out of whack. [29,30]

The reason for this disparity is the huge overconsumption of commercially processed oils. These oils are not only "death oils" (as you're now aware), they upset the ratio of EFAs your body should be receiving every day, which is also not good.

So here's how to get your EFA ratio right and reap the full benefits of these powerful nutrients...

EPO...

I believe the best source of both omega-6 and omega-3 essential fatty acids is evening primrose oil (EPO).

Known as "the good oil," EPO has been valued for centuries and in my opinion should be labelled as one of the greatest preventative supplements ever!

Evening primrose oil is a rich source of both linoleic acid (LA) and alpha-linolenic acid (ALA) – and also contains high amounts of crucial gamma-linolenic acid (GLA) for prostaglandin production. It's been well documented for its ability to lower cholesterol levels, high blood pressure and triglyceride levels rapidly without causing any adverse effects.

EPO can also be of particular benefit to people suffering from multiple sclerosis, hyperactivity and obesity. More recently, it's been shown to help women with pre-menstrual discomfort. [30]

In addition to consuming evening primrose oil, it's also a good idea to eat oily fish such as salmon, tuna, sardines, mackerel or trout two to three times a week. These are all excellent sources of the omega-3 essential fatty acids EPA and DHA. If you don't eat fish then taking a quality fish oil or krill oil supplement is a viable option.

Green leafy vegetables (especially wheat grass) are all good sources of alpha-linolenic acid, which the body uses to make essential EPA and DHA.

I also recommend going to your local health food store or visiting the health section of your supermarket and buying some hemp, pumpkin, sunflower, flax seeds (linseeds), and almonds (organic if possible). Grind them up with a coffee grinder and keep them in a dark, airtight container in the fridge. These can then be sprinkled on foods such as pasta, rice, vegetables, fruits, yogurt, breakfast cereals, or anything you like. Alternatively, you can buy an LSA mix that contains linseeds, sunflower seeds and almonds ground up. These mixtures are an excellent source of EFAs and other vital nutrients.

Benefits of Essential Fatty Acid Therapy...

Studies have consistently shown that essential fatty acids can help improve a wide variety of health conditions. These conditions range from acne and other skin disorders to assisting with proper weight management.

Evening primrose oil is an important part of EFA therapy. Amazingly, between the late 1970's and early 1990's, over 250 scientific papers were produced on the health-giving properties of evening primrose oil.

Expect to consume evening primrose oil and other EFA containing foods for at least eight weeks before seeing any significant health improvements. [30]

EFAs (evening primrose oil being a vital source) are able to help with the following conditions:

Acne:

Acne affects many people, particularly between the ages of twelve and twenty-four. It results when the sebaceous glands in the skin "clog up" with the oil that's normally used to lubricate the skin. Bacteria then begin to multiply in these glands causing inflammation.

Adolescence is when we're most susceptible to acne as the hormones that activate oil production are at their peak during these years.

Evening primrose oil can help acne sufferers by supplying gamma-linolenic acid, which is needed for skin repair and rejuvenation. Studies show when EPO is combined with zinc (contained in colloidal minerals and wheat grass) results are even more favorable. Junk foods that contain sugar, refined carbohydrates or refined oils need to be eliminated for best results as well.

It's also interesting to note that people such as the Canadian Eskimos never experienced acne or pimples until they began to include our Westernized "junk food" in their diets. That certainly tells you something doesn't it? [30]

Cancer:

Ongoing research has consistently proven that high-fat diets and cancer are *strongly* linked. Certainly not all fats of course, only the "bad fats" discussed earlier.

These particular fats upset normal prostaglandin metabolism, which researchers believe contribute to cancer development. A lack of gamma-linolenic acid (GLA) results in the body's inability to produce enough of the prostaglandin E1 (PGE1), which has also been linked to the development of certain types of cancers. [29,30]

The fact is *all* of us have the potential to get cancer everyday of our lives. What prevents this from occurring is our immune system, which is designed to eradicate any wayward cells so they don't multiply unrestrained and cause damage. If the immune system is not functioning correctly though, these abnormal cells are able to reproduce freely, resulting in tumor development.

So it's critical that our immune system always remains in peak condition. And what better way to do this than consume powerful "immune boosting" supplements such as wheat grass powder, colloidal minerals and evening primrose oil. Of course, evening primrose oil plays an important role in cancer prevention because it contains the all important gamma-linolenic acid, which has been found to have anti-tumor properties. [29,30]

Diabetes:

This horrible disease can cause many serious complications such as heart disease, blindness, kidney failure and limb amputations resulting from poor circulation.

In simple terms, Type 1 diabetes occurs when the pancreas fails to produce insulin and is marked by excess sugar in the blood and urine.

With Type 2 diabetes the pancreas produces plenty of insulin, but the body is unable to make use of it.

Because of our poor eating habits and the fact that the foods we consume today lack nutritional quality, diabetes has now become rampant amongst society.

It's known to strike any age group and symptoms include excessive thirst, frequent urination, dizziness and sugar intolerance. [29,30]

In the chapter on minerals, I spoke about how vital both chromium and vanadium are to diabetics for regulating normal insulin activity (and how vanadium will replace insulin in adult-onset diabetes). Well, in addition to consuming these important minerals, further studies have shown that evening primrose oil can also be beneficial for diabetics because it helps the body make PGE1, which has been found to mimic insulin and produce insulin-like actions! [29,30]

Obesity:

Essential fatty acids help increase the body's energy output and stimulate metabolism - assisting in weight loss and fat reduction. They break up and "dissolve" body fat and aid in the removal of hard fats (the most stubborn).

EFAs also increase the activity of brown fat, which helps the body burn fat rather than storing the excess calories as fatty tissue. Gamma-linolenic acid (found in evening primrose oil) is the main substance that stimulates brown fat metabolism.

In a study on EFAs and obesity, overweight people were given supplemental evening primrose oil every day as a part of their diet. After four weeks tests showed a substantial increase in brown fat activity, and as a result, all participants lost significant amounts of weight. [29,30]

Another Cause of Obesity...

And while I'm on the subject of obesity, I want to talk about a little-known condition called pica. This misdiagnosed condition (most doctors don't even believe it exists) affects a large majority of the population and is actually one of the main causes of obesity.

Pregnant women are renowned for getting pica, hence why many mothers-to-be will wake up during the night craving weird food combinations such as pickles and ice cream, peanut butter and jelly, sausages and jam, even pork or beef jerky with ice cream (some of the most popular).

What's happening in this instance is the growing fetus is sucking valuable nutrients, particularly minerals and trace elements, from the mother's body. She continues to eat more food in different combinations to try and replenish the supply (this is all happening on an unconscious level), but the problem is, eating foods that are nutrient-dead only causes more cravings and a substantial gain in weight.

Children can also suffer from pica. If you've ever caught your child eating from the kitty litter box or eating dirt from the sand pit, you now know why (if you didn't already). The same thing is happening here; the body is craving nutrients, particularly minerals, so it's trying to satisfy that craving. [1,9,14]

My guess is around 90% (or more) of the population today suffers from pica in varying degrees. Remember, there's barely any nutrients left in our foods, especially refined and processed foods, so people are eating more to try and satisfy their body's need for these essential nutrients. It doesn't happen of course, so they continue to eat (junk food is a popular choice as it fills the hole quickly) and so the vicious cycle continues.

Funnily enough, the snack food industry actually has a name for pica. They call it "the munchies!"

The good news is if you do suffer from pica then you'll find that within 12 months of taking in all 90 essential nutrients your food cravings will naturally start to disappear and weight loss will happen easily. [1,9,14]

Premenstrual Syndrome (PMS):

PMS is a condition that affects many women, mostly under the age of forty. It's caused by the body's imbalance of certain hormones

– mainly an overproduction of estrogen and lack of progesterone. This imbalance results in many uncomfortable side effects including irritability, anxiety, depression, mental sluggishness, cramps and fluid retention.

It's now been discovered that women who suffer with PMS are actually low in prostaglandins, especially PGE1. Evening primrose oil has brought overwhelming relief to thousands of PMS sufferers because it contains GLA, which helps to balance prostaglandin and hormone levels naturally. [29,30]

In addition to this, studies and online surveys show that PMS sufferers usually consume more bad saturated fats, trans-fatty acids, refined carbohydrates and processed dairy products than what non-sufferers do. These foods are known to exacerbate the symptoms of PMS significantly. [29,30]

Auto-immune Disorders:

These include diseases such as rheumatoid arthritis, asthma, psoriasis, eczema, multiple sclerosis, ulcerative colitis, Raynaud's disease and migraines.

T-cells are the cells in our body that make sure the immune system only attacks foreign invaders, not our own cells. Auto-immune diseases are believed to occur when this system fails and the body begins to turn on itself and attack its own cells.

Because prostaglandins affect so many of the body's immune and inflammatory responses, including the action of T-cells, maintaining healthy levels is vital in the fight against auto-immune diseases. [30]

Evening primrose oil is extremely beneficial for people suffering from auto-immune disorders as it contains the raw materials for the body to produce prostaglandins naturally. With regards to multiple sclerosis, European researchers have reported a 30% success rate for MS patients using evening primrose oil! [30]

Other Health Problems Linked to an EFA Deficiency...

There are numerous other ailments that are the result of essential fatty acid deficiencies - many of which are caused by prostaglandin imbalances.

Some of these include: fibrocystic breast disease, endometriosis, prostate disorders, infertility, depression, and skin disorders such as rosacea and dandruff.

EFA supplementation can help immensely with all of these, especially evening primrose oil, which is considered one of the most successful treatments. [29,30]

* * *

This concludes the chapter on essential fatty acids.

Now we not only know why EFAs are so important to us, we also understand why we must avoid the "bad fats" as much as possible if we're going to enjoy good health.

The next chapter is on the food that has been hailed as "one of nature's greatest health gifts."

Wheatgrass truly is the perfect food for our overall health, well-being and longevity program.

Let's find out why researchers right around the world are constantly "singing its praises!"

C H A P T E R 8

In this chapter, although I make reference to wheatgrass, this also includes the green shoots of other cereal grasses such as barley, oats and rye.

Nutritionally, they're all identical. They are, however, very different from the mature seed grains of these plants (i.e. those found in breakfast cereals), which do not have the same nutritional value as the young shoots of cereal grasses. And in case you're wondering, the young shoots of cereal grass DO NOT contain any gluten.

Natures Truly Astonishing "Miracle Food"...

Considered by many to be "a gift from above," wheatgrass is a potent food that has been valued since ancient times for its health giving properties.

The Bible makes numerous references to cereal grasses testifying to their healing benefits. The Book of Daniel in the Old Testament tells of how a sick and dying King Nebuchadnezzar II of Babylon (605-562 B.C.) ate nothing but "grasses" for seven years and attributed this to his restored health, allowing him to continue ruling and serving his kingdom.

Ancient Oriental and Middle Eastern people, once known for their longevity, were said to consume wheat and barley grass daily. [28]

Today, cereal grasses are having somewhat of a comeback, mainly due to the research that's been conducted since the late 1920's. This research has continued to confirm and validate the health and therapeutic benefits of these incredible plants.

The Perfect Food for Health

Science has deemed wheatgrass the most nutritious of all plant foods. After more than eighty years of extensive research, no other plant has come close to matching its nutritional value.

In fact, wheatgrass is such a nutritionally complete food that one could survive and flourish on consuming nothing *but* wheatgrass!

It's an excellent source of all the essential vitamins and amino acids, along with many of the major minerals. It also contains the essential fatty acid alpha-linolenic acid, which the body uses to make EPA and DHA. [31]

Not only is wheatgrass rich in the essential nutrients we need, it contains the ***perfect*** amounts and ratios of these essential nutrients.

Well known for his ongoing research into barley grass, Dr Yoshihide Hagiwara wrote: "*My research has shown that the green leaves of the embryonic barley plant contain the most prolific balanced supply of nutrients that exist on earth in a single source.*" [12]

This "balanced supply" increases the potency of wheatgrass as ***all nutrients work in synergy with each other.***

For instance, calcium and Vitamin B6 are needed for the body to absorb Vitamin B12. B12 is then used for the activation of folic acid.

Another example of this synergistic action is vitamin C helping with the absorption of calcium and iron. Iron is then needed for the body to convert beta-carotene to Vitamin A (this is yet another example of why we must obtain our daily nutrition from natural foods like wheatgrass, rather than synthetic multivitamin and mineral tablets which do not produce the same effect). [28]

So the balanced supply and synergistic action of nutrients contained in wheatgrass make it a food with *super powerful* health-building properties!

Important "Food Factors" in Cereal Grasses

Another remarkable discovery made by researchers of wheatgrass and other cereal grasses is the "unidentified food factors" they contain. These food factors have been shown to provide a vast array of health, growth and fertility benefits to humans and animals.

In one experiment, performed at UCLA Berkeley, Dr Cannon and his fellow researchers discovered that when guinea pigs were fed a normal stock ration plus high levels of synthetic nutrients, their health deteriorated rapidly. Even when standard food supplements such as brewer's yeast, liver extract and wheat germ were included in the animal's diets, they barely improved and often died. However, the introduction of cereal grasses caused a dramatic recovery and re-stimulated growth in the animals. [28]

It's understood the cereal grasses supplied powerful "hidden benefits" which were not attributable to any of the known nutrients. Even to this day, some of the special food factors and hidden benefits contained in the young shoots of cereal grasses have still not been identified!

The Healing Power of Chlorophyll

Chlorophyll, the green pigment in plants, is one of the "food factors" in wheatgrass and other cereal grasses.

Although it's not classed as a nutrient, chlorophyll's potent health and healing benefits are certainly well recognized.

Known as a "blood-builder" its molecular structure is similar to hemoglobin - the protein molecule that carries oxygen in the blood.

Many of the nutrients that build and sustain the blood (Vitamin C, Vitamin K, folic acid, beta-carotene, calcium, iron, Vitamin B6 and protein) are contained in foods high in chlorophyll.

Chlorophyll is extremely important for building strong red blood cells and preventing the condition known as rouleaux (when this occurs the red blood cells stick together in chains instead of moving about freely). Rouleaux blood is sick blood, which in turn causes lethargy and many debilitating health problems. [28]

A study on "blood building," researched by biochemist and nutritionist, Dr Ziema McDonell, from the Nutritional Health and Information Centre in Sydney, showed when wheatgrass was given to all different types of people, it was far superior and faster at building up the blood than any of the conventional treatments that were usually employed. [32]

Remember this... healthy blood is vital for the supplying of oxygen and nutrients to the cells and the removal of carbon dioxide and waste material from the cells. Any deterioration of this process can pose a *serious threat* to our overall health and well-being!

More Health Benefits of Chlorophyll...

Chlorophyll is a powerful deodorant and will rid the body of any unwanted odors. It offers protection from the ingestion of toxic chemicals as well as helping with the elimination (chelation) of harmful toxins from the body.

Chlorophyll has been well documented for its ability to accelerate wound healing by stimulating new cell growth whilst limiting dangerous bacterial growth. The topical use of chlorophyll on any type of wound is tremendously beneficial and has actually saved many limbs from amputation. [28]

In addition to this, overwhelming evidence has now proven that chlorophyll and the nutrients contained in green foods *protect the body against radiation and the cancer-causing effects of carcinogens*. Chlorophyll has also been shown to reduce the damaging effects of carcinogens in regards to their ability to cause gene mutations (mutations to our genes can cause many disastrous health problems such as birth defects, cystic fibrosis and cancer).[28]

Other studies have found chlorophyll effective in the healing of peptic ulcers and pancreatitis, along with colon diseases such as spastic colitis, sigmoiditis and ulcerative colitis. Chlorophyll also promotes bowel regularity and is renowned for helping ease joint pain and inflammation.

And the good news is... wheatgrass is an extremely rich source of chlorophyll!

Cereal Grasses Are Also Packed With Valuable Live Enzymes...

What are enzymes and why do we need them?

In a nutshell, enzymes are substances (catalysts) that enable two proteins to come together and react with each other with minimum effort, which means they also reduce the amount of energy that would normally be required for this process to take place.

Certain proteins in the body are needed for chemical reactions to take place. Enzymes not only make this life sustaining task possible; they help speed up the process significantly.

Enzymes are essential for just about every bodily function – so essential in fact that we wouldn't even be able to move (or exist) for that matter without them!

They not only control our state of health, but our lifespan as well.

We Only Have a Limited Amount of "Enzyme Energy"

Scientists believe that each of us only has a given amount of enzyme energy at birth, which must last for our entire lives. This means that if we use up this supply prematurely, our lives are shortened.

According to enzyme researcher, Dr Edward Howell, one way this primarily occurs is when we eat too much of what I call "enzyme dead" foods (refined and processed foods, overcooked foods).

The problem with these foods is the enzymes in our bodies have to do all the work to break down the proteins, starches and fats - which means we eventually become enzyme deficient, even by middle age. Once this occurs our bodies cannot be supplied with the vital nutrients they need in a form that can be absorbed.

Other factors such as age (digestive enzymes diminish as we grow older), disease and stress can also result in the body being unable to maintain adequate levels of enzymes. [12]

If on the other hand, we eat plenty of raw vegetables, fruits, and seeds, our bodies will not only be supplied with the essential enzymes they need, but the live enzymes contained in these "live foods" will help breakdown and digest our meal rather than our own enzymes. This means we are able to reserve our enzyme supply, and theoretically, live longer.

Low Enzyme Levels Weaken Your Immunity

Low enzyme levels will also cause your immune system to become severely weakened, leaving you open to many serious illnesses and diseases including arthritis, diabetes, heart disease, cancer, obesity and various allergies.

One study showed that patients who died from debilitating diseases such as diabetes, liver disease and cancer had very low levels of enzymes in their pancreas compared to patients who were considered healthy when they died. [12]

Diseases like cancer not only rob the body of important nutrients, they also prohibit the manufacture of enzymes.

Now more than ever, it's **critical** that we protect our enzyme supply by consuming plenty of "live foods" that are rich in valuable live enzymes. [12]

As a final note; many health-conscious people believe that live foods contain a "living energy" that gives vitality and a sense of aliveness to those who eat them. Scientists would be hard pressed to measure this, but raw food advocates, such as Dr Gabriel Cousens (acclaimed author of the million copy bestseller, *Spiritual Nutrition)*, swear by it.

Thankfully, powdered cereal grasses are a *potent* "live food" practically bursting with precious live enzymes!

Research and Healing Stories...

As I said earlier, wheatgrass and other cereal grasses have been extensively studied for well over eighty years.

Much of this research was intensive until the late 1950's when synthetic vitamin and mineral pills became available.

Research then slowed dramatically until the late 1960s when Dr Ann Wigmore began researching and rediscovering the therapeutic value of cereal grasses...

After her health began to deteriorate, she started consuming the young shoots of wheatgrass every day - which she grew herself at home.

Not only did she regain her health within weeks, her energy levels increased dramatically and she was able to recover from a serious colitis problem that was unable to be treated successfully medically.

Dr Wigmore then started giving wheatgrass juice to her frail and sick elderly neighbors. She reported that after only a few weeks these people were out of their beds and leading active lives. [28]

In 1968, Dr Wigmore founded the *Hippocrates Health Institute* in Boston, which was designed to treat patients with chronic degenerative diseases using wheatgrass and other raw green foods. Amazingly, people were cured of diseases that were considered "terminal" by their doctors.

Many cancer patients recovered from the disease after being told that nothing more could be done for them. One such person was Eydie Mae Hunsberger, who tells of her astonishing recovery in her bestselling book *How I Conquered Cancer Naturally*.

Dr Wigmore discovered that cereal grasses contain powerful anti-cancer substances, particularly abscisic acid and laetrile (vitamin B17), along with chlorophyll and other anti-cancer nutrients about to be discussed.

From her experiences with her patients at the *Hippocrates Health Institute*, Dr Wigmore believes the young shoots of cereal grasses and other chlorophyll-rich plants are an effective and safe treatment for many of the common ailments that plague society today, some of which include; diabetes mellitus, high blood pressure, obesity, cancer, asthma, liver and pancreatic problems, constipation, hemorrhoids, gastritis, ulcers, fatigue, halitosis, body odor, eczema and other skin problems. [28]

Japanese Doctor Also Discovers the Benefits of Wheat Grass...

During the late 1960s, another doctor also began to research and study the health and therapeutic benefits of cereal grasses – in particular, barley grass.

Dr Yoshihide Hagiwara, a Japanese medical doctor and research pharmacist, developed a number of chronic health problems at the age of 38.

After trying unsuccessfully to restore his health through the use of modern drugs and megadoses of synthetic vitamins and minerals, he found improvement through Chinese herbal remedies and a radical change in diet.

Hagiwara then began a search to find *the* most beneficial and health-promoting food available. After ten years of research on over 300 green plants at all stages of maturity, he declared that *"the leaves of the cereal grasses provide the nearest thing to the perfect food that this planet offers."* [12,28]

Dr Hagiwara, along with his colleagues in Japan and America, continued to study the benefits of barley grass, consistently finding more and more evidence of this food's astonishing health building properties. Many of these benefits have been discussed and documented in the best-selling books *Green Leaves of Barley* by Dr Mary Ruth Swope and *Cereal Grass — Nature's Greatest Health Gift* by Ronald Seibold, M.S.

More Remarkable Research Results

There have certainly been some impressive results published from various studies on cereal grasses and other green foods.

For example, Japanese researchers found that wheatgrass significantly lowers serum cholesterol – due mainly to its unique ability to block the intestinal absorption of excess cholesterol. [12,28]

In 1984, Japanese researchers isolated two important proteins in wheatgrass (P4-D1 and D1-G1), which may be some of the unidentified food factors revealed earlier. P4-D1 was found to protect the body's cells from harmful cancer-causing substances and ultraviolet radiation, which researchers believe may be linked to its ability to stimulate DNA repair. [12,28]

A recently discovered isoflavonoid in wheatgrass has been shown to exert strong antioxidant activity and inhibit lipid peroxidation (a harmful process that occurs in the body during the digestion of the "bad fats" discussed previously). Another flavonoid in wheatgrass, 2-O-GIV, has incredibly strong anti-allergic, anti-inflammatory and antioxidant activity. [12,28]

In 1994, Japanese and American researchers identified the molecules in wheatgrass responsible for the stimulation of growth hormone and lactation hormone in women, confirming wheatgrass's benefit to pregnant and lactating women. Cereal grasses have also been shown to increase fertility in both men and women and assist with the growth of lactobacilli and other "friendly" intestinal bacteria (acting as an effective prebiotic). [12,28]

Stomach Ulcers, Skin Disorders and Cancer...

Back in the 1950's, cereal grasses were found to promote the rapid healing of peptic ulcers and many skin diseases.

Research during 1979-1980 indicated that grasses not only contain some extremely powerful cancer preventative properties, they may even be able to reverse the effects of this deadly disease. [28]

A report published in the *Journal of the National Cancer Institute* affirmed that patients hospitalised with bowel cancer have a history of consuming fewer green vegetables than patients who are free of the disease. Studies show that eating green vegetables greatly reduce one's risk of developing stomach, ovarian and cervical cancers.

In addition to these, green foods offer some protection for smokers from lung cancer...

Italian researchers discovered that smokers who consume green vegetables and carrots are far less likely to develop lung cancer than smokers who seldom eat these vegetables. This is mainly due to the high amount of beta-carotene they contain, but other substances and nutrients in these foods certainly contribute to this protective effect. [28]

So these are just some of the many research results produced over the past eighty years confirming cereal grasses' value as a highly nutritious food!

Cereal Grasses Are Powerful Detoxifiers

Toxins are harmful substances that we are all exposed to every day of our lives. In actual fact, even normal bodily functions such as breathing and digestion produce toxins. We are also exposed to thousands of toxic chemicals as a result of the contaminated air we breathe, water we drink and food we eat.

If these poisons are not "flushed out" every day they begin to quickly build-up and cause many unwanted health problems including lethargy, chronic fatigue, obesity, hormonal dysfunction, allergies and decreased immune function - along with diseases such as cancer, diabetes, leukemia, Alzheimer's, arthritis, and heart disease, to name a few. [12]

For us to fully understand the destructive damage that toxins do to our bodies, we must first understand where this damage begins....

All body tissues (including skin, bone, connective tissue and organs) consist of cells. For us to maintain excellent health and live to our genetic potential, each cell in our body must remain in peak condition.

For this to happen, cells must be supplied with the essential nutrients, to not only nourish them, but allow the constant removal of all harmful chemicals and toxins. If this doesn't occur then our cells degenerate, ***resulting in degeneration of the body.***

So the damage toxins inflict on us begins at the cellular level, the very core of the human body.

Free Radicals and Antioxidants

Most people today have heard of free radicals and antioxidants - but what *exactly* are they?

Free radicals are basically "aggressive molecules" that are produced as a result of our normal metabolic processes and from the accumulation of toxins and chemicals within the body.

These "bad guys" go around messing up the functions of our healthy cells. They indiscriminately kill healthy cells, destroy essential enzymes and produce toxic chemicals that disturb cellular membranes.

Free radicals are associated with the aging process and even death itself! [12,25]

Research by Professor Hannes Staehelin, head of the Geriatric Clinic at the University of Basel in Switzerland, revealed that memory deterioration in relation to aging is closely linked to free radical damage. It was discovered that neurons located in brain cells are severely affected by free radicals. This "destruction" causes massive disturbances to memory and cognitive functions. Professor Staehelin stated that "antioxidants appear to protect brain neurons from damage." [33]

Free radicals also damage the DNA structure of a cell causing mutations to that cell. Once this occurs, the mutated cell will <u>only</u> reproduce the altered version. (This is the beginning of diseases such as cancer). Mutated cells can also cause would-be parents to pass on "hereditary" diseases to their unborn children. [12,25]

Antioxidants, on the other hand, are the protectors and healers.

Their job is to prevent, and when required, repair the damage that's been done by the rampaging free radicals. These guys basically go around "cleaning up the mess," if you like.

It's interesting to note that our bodies do have their own natural antioxidant system, but environmental and lifestyle factors such as pollution, toxic chemicals, radiation and stress all result in excessive free radical production (known as toxic overload). As we age, our natural antioxidant system also becomes less efficient.

The only way we can effectively combat and defeat these bad guys is by taking in an adequate daily supply of high strength antioxidants!

Vitamins C, E and beta-carotene (Pro-Vitamin A), as well as selenium, zinc, manganese and copper, along with the amino acids methionine and cysteine, are all potent antioxidants (all are found abundantly in cereal grasses too by the way). [12,25]

One particular enzyme known as super-oxide dismutase (SOD), currently has researchers world-wide very excited. SOD has been hailed as one of the finest and most powerful antioxidants discovered thus far. This outstanding detoxifier plays a crucial role in protecting the body from degenerative diseases caused by free radical damage. [12, 25]

SOD's main function is to shield each cell from the destruction and deterioration caused by superoxides (free radicals), along with helping remove stubborn residual chemicals and heavy metals from the body.

Studies have shown that SOD, along with the enzyme P4-D1, can actually *repair* damaged DNA. And because they have the ability to repair human genes, including those in reproductive cells, researchers believe SOD and P4-D1 may help prevent birth defects and the passing on of genetic diseases to offspring. [12,25]

Research has also shown that super-oxide dismutase can reduce the pain and inflammation of arthritis, slow down the aging process, and greatly reduce the chances of someone developing cancer or other degenerative disease. Further studies on heart attack victims found SOD effective in the repairing of damaged heart tissue. [12,25]

An extract from research carried out by the *Science University of Tokyo* confirms the amazing power of super-oxide dismutase. Here's what it says...

This enzyme has drawn tremendous attention from biologists, biochemists and other doctors in relation to cancer and carcinogenesis. Recently the importance of SOD has been extended to the study of some genetic diseases (bloom syndrome) and immune diseases. Its use in the medical field is being considered. Young barley plants contain a large amount of active SOD. This has been studied extensively and described in earlier reports. The barley SOD could be contributing to many of the phenomena young barley has shown so far. For example, superoxides inside the cells and surrounding the cells can cause damage to DNA. Older cells and environmentally or artificially damaged cells can have higher levels of superoxide and thus create more damage to cellular DNA. Green barley contains the enzyme SOD to remove superoxides and repair damaged DNA, together with lectin-like material to reactivate cells and tissues thus re-activating them as well as aiding in recovery from disease. [34]

Thank goodness, wheat grass and other cereal grasses are a rich source of this marvellous enzyme, which has much to do with longevity!

More Potent Detoxifiers...

There are even more powerful detoxifiers contained in cereal grasses that have been found to neutralize poisonous chemicals and other harmful substances in the body.

For instance, the enzyme known as nitrate reductase is able to break down nitric-compounds from petroleum solvents, which actually make up about seventy percent of carcinogens. P4-D1 has also been found to neutralize harmful nitric-compounds, along with the chemical food preservative BHT. [12]

Reports from several researchers back in 1981 showed that wheat grass neutralizes benzpyrene – a chemical from tobacco that causes lung cancer. Further studies found wheat grass is able to neutralize two other deadly carcinogens, TRY-P1 and TRY-P2. These substances, which are 20,000 times more carcinogenic than benzpyrene, are primarily produced from char-grilling fish, red meat, sausages, etc, on open grills. [12]

Further detoxifiers contained in cereal grasses include various flavonoids, which detoxify the cells, and certain amino acids, which are able to neutralize nicotine and dissolve heavy metals such as mercury and lead. Other substances called mucopolysaccharides, as well as the enzyme catalase, are currently being investigated as a possible treatment for cancer. [12]

And once again... cereal grasses have been found to contain *rich* amounts of all of these substances!

The Importance of Dietary Fibre

The need for fibre in the diet has received increased attention in recent years, due in most part to the growing number of diseases that have now been associated with the over-consumption of refined and processed foods and the under consumption of dietary fibre.

Fibre is important for maintaining a healthy and well functioning digestive tract (stomach, small and large intestine, colon).

The organ that most people give little or no thought to is the colon - but this body part performs an essential, although unattractive function. If it's not working properly then conditions such as constipation, diarrhea, colitis, diverticulitis and irritable bowel syndrome will result. [35]

A poorly functioning colon makes a perfect breeding ground for unhealthy bacteria and parasites to reside and propagate. This causes deterioration of the bowel and the accompanying health problems.

In addition, if the colon isn't functioning correctly then this also forces dirty, toxic liquid to be recirculated back into the body. The tissues and organs then become the "waste disposal" or "dumping ground" for the toxic material that should have been eliminated. Our overall health and vitality can only suffer under these horrendous conditions.

Natural Therapist, Peter O'Hara, sums this up well:

Consider what happens to the health of a city when the waste disposal or sewerage systems are inefficient. The potential for disease increases dramatically. Disease potential is equally high when the colon does not function healthily. [35]

Lack of Fibre Increases Your Risk of Colon Cancer

In industrialized countries such as the U.S., Australia and Great Britain, colon cancer is the third most common form of cancer - yet in developing countries it's extremely rare. The reason for this is the high fibre foods (fruits, vegetables and wholegrains) these people consume compared to the high number of processed foods that are primarily eaten by Western civilisations.

It's interesting to note too that health problems such as colitis, diverticulitis and irritable bowel syndrome are virtually unheard of in most developing countries. [35]

*Studies have now been able to confirm that there is a **direct link** between colon cancer and a lack of fibre in the diet.* [35]

Fibre is important as it carries toxins out of the body, gently cleans the walls of the bowel and helps promote regular bowel movements. This process prevents carcinogens and other harmful substances from accumulating in the colon, which is believed to be the root cause of bowel cancer.

More Reasons for Dietary Fibre

Recent research into diabetes has found that dietary fibre is able to decrease glucose levels in the blood and help to alleviate insulin dependence for diabetics.

It also lowers blood pressure (with no harmful side effects) and helps build up the supply of much needed "friendly" bacteria in the colon. [28,35]

Fibre is also an excellent weight loss and slimming aid...

It has a unique water-binding action that produces a feeling of fullness in the stomach, so the overall amount of food and calories consumed is naturally reduced. In addition, fibre itself has zero calories, which further benefits anyone on a weight control/weight loss program.

The old saying that fibre "keeps you regular" is certainly true, however, it should not be confused with any type of laxative. These products actually promote laziness in the bowel (for instance, the common laxative cascara rushes the digestion process and prevents nutrient absorption), whereas fibre actually helps with the digestion and elimination process in a natural way. [35]

What is the Best Source of Dietary Fibre?

As you've probably already guessed, dehydrated cereal grasses contain rich amounts of this vital nutrient, as a recent health article on the importance of fibre points out:

One of the biggest injustices we can inflict on our bodies is to deprive it of natural fibre. The digestive tract needs this to keep it working properly by toning it, keeping it oxygenated and maintaining the friendly flora. Natural fibre provides us with sustained energy because it is a complex carbohydrate. The best source of this is the naturally occurring fibre in tender young green plant life, such as in shoots of green barley and wheat. This fibre contains the mineral spectrum of the plant and many of the vitamins. This type of fibre is quite different from the husks of seeds and grains, although these are a necessary component of a good diet also, but only as part of the whole food that we ingest. [36]

So, here's the bottom line (pardon the pun) … without fibre, the colon and the rest of our digestive system suffers. If our digestive system suffers, our health suffers!

The Remarkable Healing Power of Wheat Grass...

As a result of my own personal research into wheat grass, I discovered that not only are there many people enjoying the wonderful health benefits this food provides, but many others have also overcome serious and life threatening diseases and afflictions from the daily intake of wheat grass.

Some were even considered "incurable" by doctors using conventional methods, yet by feeding the body "nature's miracle food," it was able to completely repair and heal itself.

I would like to share with you one such story, which I believe will give hope to many people who might be suffering from a serious disease or ailment and may have lost all hope of recovery.

It's about a wonderful Australian man - Les Dyne...

Back in 1982, Les was a respected and high class lawyer operating out of a plush office and earning a very healthy income for himself. With the world at his feet, life was seemingly good for Les. That was until he started to feel "off" and began losing weight. After resisting for many months, Les finally visited his M.D. to find out what was wrong.

After numerous tests, Doctors discovered a large cancerous tumor in his pelvic area and eight inches of the pelvic bone had actually wasted away. The muscles in his left leg had also begun to degenerate.

Worryingly, Les's cancer development was already stage 4 (the most serious) and doctors strongly suggested that the left leg and pelvis be amputated immediately.

For Les, however, this wasn't an option. Instead, he decided to pursue the usual conventional treatments - chemotherapy and radiation.

He was told that it could take six to twelve months before he could expect to see real positive results. Astonishingly, he endured the horrendous chemotherapy cycles for three years, as well as six weeks of daily radiation treatment - only to find that after all of this the tumor had barely even shrunk!

With the doctors unable to do anything more for him, and basically sent home to die, Les decided to look for another alternative to help him overcome the disease.

He came to the conclusion that trying to fight the cancer with chemicals and radiation was in fact doing him more harm than good.

Les began to research natural recovery methods and discovered that when the body is fed live organic nutrition, it's able to cleanse, repair and regenerate itself.

He knew that for him to recover, giving his body the right nutrients, co-factors and antioxidants everyday was a must. As Les says: *"We wouldn't give a builder the job of repairing our home without the right materials, yet we expect our body to do it all the time".*

This research is what led him to the nutritional marvel that is wheat grass.

Les began consuming twelve teaspoons of powdered organic wheat grass (barley grass) everyday and noticed positive results almost immediately.

Within two weeks his energy levels rose dramatically and he was able to enjoy a sense of well being that he hadn't felt in many years.

Amazingly, after only three months the pelvic bone had actually regenerated (the x-rays were able to clearly show this) and within six months doctors could find no trace of the tumor! [37]

With the supplying of correct nutrients, live enzymes and other important "food factors," Les's body was able to heal and repair itself within a very short period of time. The doctors, of course, labelled it a "miracle".

So how is Les doing today? Well, it's now been over forty years since his initial diagnosis and Les is still fighting fit. And instead of going back to his well paid law practice, he now spends his time educating others on the importance of good nutrition and health practices. He also spends his time educating farmers on the need for more sustainable agriculture (i.e., putting minerals back into the soil, farming without the use of pesticides, non GMO's, etc.)

While Les was trying to fight his cancer, he made a commitment that if he found a way to beat the disease, he would spend the rest of his life helping others do the same. He still continues to honour that commitment today!

Les is Not the Only One...

What I find remarkable about Les's story is that all he did was supplement his diet with powdered barley grass. That's all he did! And he cured himself of the big C.

But Les is not alone. There are hundreds of similar stories around the world from people who've managed to overcome life threatening diseases through the daily consumption of green foods such as cereal grasses, chlorella and spirulina.

Danny McDonald from Ireland is probably the most famous. This guy completely healed himself from stage 4 stomach cancer (one of the deadliest) through the daily intake of wheatgrass. Gisela Tomlinson and Cuiva Smith are two other well known women who also managed to cure their cancers with wheatgrass (and Gisela went on to live to be 96 years of age).

These people, with the help of potent green "super foods" such as wheat grass and barley grass, were able to overcome what some would say were impossible odds. They all know, however, that once they discovered the wonderful healing power of cereal grasses, the odds were no longer impossible, but were now stacked heavily in *their* favour!

"The Best and Most Lasting Cures are Those Which Allow the Body to Heal Itself"

Ronald L. Seibold, M.S. [28]

Juiced or Dehydrated Powders… Which are Better?

If we're going to enjoy the full health benefits that wheat grass offers, I believe it's important that we choose the most potent form for maximum results.

There are two methods used for the processing of wheat grass – dehydration and juicing. Dehydration has been found to be the superior method. [28,38]

When the plant is dried at body temperature, precious live enzymes and vitamins are retained and not destroyed by heat. When the wheat grass is finally ground down to a powder, this must also be done at low temperatures so as to protect the valuable nutrients.

A major benefit of dehydrated wheat grass is the retainment of the whole leaf, which means the mineral rich fibre is also preserved. With the dehydration method there's also a minimal amount of processing involved and the wheat grass is not denatured or altered in any way. This means it still retains all of its essential health-building qualities.

"Juicing" on the other hand, is the method where only the juice of the plant is extracted and retained.

This type of processing involves several procedures in order to make the juice ready for human consumption, including the adding of maltodextrin (maltodextrin is a highly processed powdered syrup made from plant starch when it's heated and treated with sulphuric acid). This substance is actually classified as a refined sugar.

What concerns me about juiced wheat grass is the denaturing that occurs during processing. This is not the way nature intended us to consume this vital food.

Another major problem with juiced wheat grass is because only the juice is extracted, it doesn't contain any of the valuable fibre of the plant (this is thrown away).

Comparative analysis of juiced and dehydrated wheat grasses clearly shows the nutritional superiority of the dehydrated products. They have nearly three times more chlorophyll, four times more copper and boron, four times more beta-carotene, seven times more iron and almost twice as much zinc as the juiced varieties. [28,38]

Dehydrated wheat grass also contains more amino acids and has the added advantage of being packed with fibre.

As a final note, it's important that the dehydrated cereal grass product we buy is organically grown in mineral rich soils (unfortunately not all of them are).

Of course, it also needs to be completely natural and free of any additives.

It certainly pays to shop around and ask questions in order to find the best quality product. Remember – your health depends on it!

* * *

Well, that brings to an end this chapter on wheat grass.

I think you'll agree that the health and healing properties of this wonderful food are nothing short of amazing.

I hope you now understand just how necessary wheat grass and other cereal grasses are for us if we're going to enjoy living long and healthy lives. They've certainly stood the test of time, wouldn't you say?

The next chapter is on the importance of probiotics (and prebiotics).

These good gut bacteria play a crucial role in nutrient absorption and protecting the body from germ invasion and disease. In fact, Hippocrates once said... _"All disease first begins in the gut,"_ and these friendly flora are the number one organisms that help keep our guts healthy!

So, let's find out some important facts about these intriguing little creatures, shall we?...

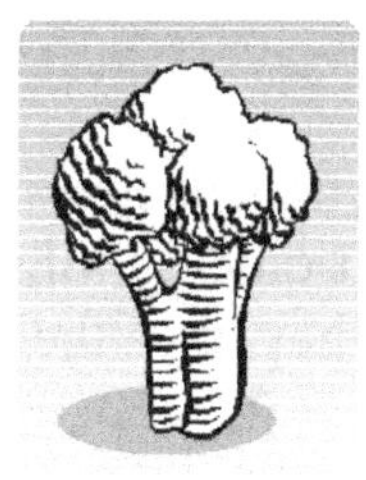

In the chapter on longevity, I gave you a brief introduction to the lactobacillus bacteria and why the fermenting of foods contributes to the longevity that certain cultures enjoy. In this chapter, I would like to explain in more detail just why these beneficial flora are so vital.

The Most Important Health Discovery of the Last Millennium...

It's fascinating to think that every one of us has trillions of little microorganisms living inside our bodies, all coexisting with each other.

One particular type of microorganism, the lactobacillus bacteria, perform many crucial functions and are essential for our overall health and vitality.

Ingesting foods that contain these "friendly" bacteria allows them to grow and thrive in the digestive system and gain dominance over the "unfriendly" bacteria.

If this doesn't occur - and the unhealthy bacteria take control - disease, infections and other serious ailments soon begin to stamp their authority.

The beauty of the lactobacillus bacteria is it produces a powerful antibiotic type substance that quickly kills harmful bacteria, fungi, viruses and protozoa before they have the chance to wreak havoc.

So you could say it's one of the ultimate internal protectors. [39,40]

Meet the Family...

There are several types of probiotics that form part of the lactobacillus family... Acidophilus, Bifidus, Casei, Bulgaricus, Fermenti and Lactis.

Acidophilus is the major form of lactobacillus bacteria and is primarily found in the intestines and vagina. They live and thrive on the walls of these body parts, acting as a first line of defence to protect the body from candida and other germ invasions.

Interestingly, candida and various other germs and bacteria also permanently reside in the body (you can't get rid of them all completely), but as long as there's a healthy supply of friendly bacteria, they won't pose any threat. If, however, the good bacteria are compromised, room is then made for these unhealthy organisms to propagate and take over - which they do so very quickly. [39,40]

So basically, as long as healthy levels of probiotics are maintained, these bad guys will simply pass through the body and not even bother trying to take up residence!

Why Gut Health is a Top Priority

70% of your immune system is actually located in your gut, so a healthy gut means a healthy and strong immune system. And probiotics are the *crucial* ingredient needed for overall gut health. In fact, the lactobacillus bacteria play an essential role in maintaining the health of the *entire* gastrointestinal tract - not just the gut.

Low levels of these beneficial bacteria mean harmful substances are unable to be excreted from the body quickly and efficiently. This in turn creates some extremely unhealthy conditions (such as the ones discussed in the section on fibre) and results in foul smelling gas and stools caused by the bad bacterial cultures.

In countries such as Finland, where they consume high amounts of foods rich in acidophilus and other friendly bacteria, they have low rates of colon cancer. [39]

The lactobacillus bacteria are also important for the digestion and assimilation of foods. If levels are low, our bodies are not able to utilize the vital nutrients we need. Inadequate levels contribute to other digestive disorders such as constipation, heartburn and bloating as well. [39,40]

The Detrimental Factors...

There are various environmental factors and lifestyle habits that affect the normal balance of healthy intestinal flora. Some of these include: exposure to chemicals and pollution, excessive sugar and fat intake, lack of fibre in the diet, use of antihistamines and oral contraceptives, overuse of aspirin and pain killers, excessive coffee intake, stress - and the main one, overuse of antibiotics. [39,40]

As a matter of fact, in regards to antibiotics and healthy gut bacteria, many gastro-intestinal specialists are now extremely concerned as the high amount of antibiotics being prescribed to patients these days are destroying the good bacteria in their digestive systems - which in turn is leaving these people exposed to some very serious and dangerous health problems!

I think many medical practitioners really do underestimate just how vital these friendly bacteria are to our health and well-being. If they did understand, surely they would recommend **all** of their patients on medications consume plenty of lactobacillus rich foods and take a high quality probiotic supplement every day?

Best Foods for Propagating Good Gut Bacteria

There are several ways in which to obtain and grow a healthy supply of beneficial bacteria in the gut. Here's the top 3...

Yogurt: This is the most popular. Best yogurts to go with are coconut, soy, Greek, and Skyr (Icelandic) yogurts. Whichever one of these you choose, just make sure it's natural (no aspartame) and is low in sugar - or even better, contains none at all. The healthiest option is to make your own yogurt at home.

Fermented Food and Drinks: Culturing your own food and drinks is one of the best and cheapest ways to get a potent supply of lactobacillus and other friendly bacteria. Sauerkraut, kefir milk (my favorite), kefir water, tempeh, miso, kombucha, kimchi, and yes, yogurt, are the most common fermented food and drinks.

Fermenting is really not that hard once you get the hang of it. There are lots of good websites and videos out there explaining exactly how to get started and how to consistently ferment for very low cost.

Probiotic Supplements: I like to think of taking a good quality probiotic supplement as an insurance policy for your gut. By consciously putting those live lactobacilli in your mouth every day you know you're definitely getting those beneficial bacteria in a highly absorbable form... so you've got your gut covered no matter what!

You can buy probiotic supplements from any good health food store or online retailer. Even supermarkets and Chemists (drug stores) now stock them in abundance.

…The best way to make sure you get plenty of good gut bacteria everyday is of course to utilise all three methods listed. Remember this, you can NEVER overdose on probiotics and you can NEVER have too much.

In fact, the more you have the merrier!

Benefits of Lactobacillus Bacteria

Continued research into the benefits of the lactobacilli bacteria have come up with some wonderful and exciting results. Here's just a few to whet your appetite:

• Contain powerful anti-cancer and anti-tumour factors;

• Able to neutralize cancer-causing chemicals;

• Help stimulate the immune system;

• Contain strong cholesterol lowering factors;

• Shown to increase resistance to disease;

• Able to fully suppress yeast and thrush growth (candida albicans);

• Produce powerful organic and inorganic antibiotics;

•Contain anti-depressant, anti-anxiety and anti-fatigue properties;

• Produce strong anti-viral and anti-fungal substances;

• Help with the manufacture and release of B group vitamins (including vitamin B12 and folic acid) into the intestines;

- Shown to enhance the breakdown and absorption of essential food components and nutrients;

- Able to alleviate gastrointestinal problems such as constipation, flatulence and bloating;

- Shown to significantly improve calcium absorption. [16]

Ailments Helped by Probiotic Therapy...

To finish off, here's some conditions that can either be helped tremendously or completely eradicated through the recolonization of friendly bacteria. Some have already been covered, but I think it's important they be elaborated on further...

Candida Albicans

This is a nasty fungus that lives in the body, particularly in the digestive tract and vagina. As long as low levels are maintained, it will exist without causing any harm.

The problem occurs when the immune system is lowered and there aren't enough beneficial bacteria in the intestines to control the fungus yeast growth. The candida will then start to invade and colonize the cells and tissues of the body.

Once they've "taken up residence," the yeast fungi discharge candida buds and toxic chemicals into the bloodstream, which then cause a variety of health problems.

Slowly, these health problems become chronic and the immune system is unable to destroy the fungus. The body then has to suffer the persistent destructive nature of this fungus as it continues to grow and take over.

Lactobacillus acidophilus is able to completely control candida albicans. It doesn't actually kill the fungus, rather, it creates an environment where the beneficial bacteria (itself) can grow and flourish, leaving no room for the virulent candida to live. [39,40]

If you suffer with candida then all yeast containing foods must be eliminated from your diet, at least until the yeast infection is fully under control. Supplementation with a high quality probiotic supplement is also a must.

Foods that need to be omitted from the diet to control yeast fungus include: all sugar and sweets (candida feed off sugar), pasteurized milk, products containing white flour, yeast breads, beer, wine, cheese, mushrooms, all refined and processed foods, vinegar products, and junk food.

Cancer

The lactobacilli bacteria have been found to be beneficial in the prevention and treatment of cancer – particularly colon cancer. These organisms help prevent toxic substances in the colon being converted into cancer causing carcinogens. Lactobacilli stop the growth of unhealthy bacteria as well, which also produce these deadly carcinogens as a result of their excretion (disgusting I know).[39,40]

The digestive tract is constantly being exposed to harmful substances as they enter the body. When the lactobacillus bacteria are plentiful however, these substances are quickly neutralized and unable to cause harm, preventing diseases such as cancer from gaining a strangle hold.

New research has shown these beneficial bacteria also help contain the growth of cancer cells, which is yet another reason why re-establishing the intestines with a healthy supply of friendly bacteria is one more important weapon in the fight against this horrible disease. [39]

Leaky Gut Syndrome

This condition is a very common (but poorly recognized) problem affecting more and more people in society today. It results when large "gaps" form between the cells of the gut wall. These gaps or holes then allow toxins, bacteria and food to seep out.

Harmful substances such as parasites, fungi, and yes, toxins and bacteria, along with other foreign material, are normally eliminated through the digestive system. However, with leaky gut syndrome, these substances are allowed to escape and enter the bloodstream. As you can imagine, the effect this can have on one's health can be very serious and even life threatening. [40]

Another problem with leaky gut syndrome is it triggers the immune system to produce and release antibodies. These antibodies then attack the lining of the gut causing various gastrointestinal disorders such as colitis and Crohn's disease.

Other problems associated with leaky gut syndrome include rheumatoid arthritis, asthma, eczema, migraines, inflammatory bowel syndrome (IBS), liver disease, cystic fibrosis, psoriasis, lupus, food/chemical sensitivities, and immune deficiencies. [40]

The lactobacilli bacteria play an important role in the prevention and healing of leaky gut syndrome. Consuming foods rich in probiotics - as well as wheat grass and evening primrose oil - help to heal the digestive tract and rid the body of leaky gut syndrome.[40]

Constipation

Constipation affects many people but most have no idea just how much of a threat this problem can be to their health.

If the colon isn't functioning efficiently (experienced as

constipation), fecal matter remains in the bowel instead of being removed.

Harmful substances that should have been excreted are now left in the colon and converted into carcinogens. These toxins and chemicals also re-enter the bloodstream, gradually poisoning the whole body.

If this isn't enough, bacteria and parasites are also free to breed and colonize in the colon (yuck), causing further deterioration of the bowel. [39,40]

The quicker waste matter moves through the bowels, the less chance of these problems occurring. It's important that the body has one to three bowel movements a day *and* these movements be accomplished without straining. The stool should also be solid but soft, not hard like the rock of Gibraltar!

Fortunately, lactobacillus acidophilus is of great benefit to anyone suffering from constipation, as this simple study revealed...

When 194 patients with constipation were given a probiotic food containing acidophilus over 95% of them were able to cease using laxatives. The positive results remained as long as the participants continued to eat the prescribed probiotic rich food. [39,40]

Also remember that fibre from dehydrated cereal grasses, along with herbal fibre formulas, are extremely important for preventing constipation and promoting regular bowel movements. So don't forget to include these in your diet and supplementation program as well.

Diarrhea

This malady occurs when certain irritants become attached to the walls of the colon and are unable to be eliminated. In trying to dislodge and remove these irritants, the bowel forces waste matter out as fast as possible, causing diarrhea.

An imbalance of intestinal flora – namely, too many bad bacteria cultures, can cause diarrhea. Restoring the supply of beneficial bacteria to the intestines can help tremendously with this condition.[39]

In addition, fibre (again from cereal grasses and herbal fibre formulas) is also important for overcoming and preventing diarrhea as this valuable nutrient gently cleans and soothes the walls of the bowel.

Other problems associated with low levels of good gut bacteria include:

Lactose Intolerance

Lactobacillus acidophilus significantly improve the absorption of lactose. [39]

Allergies

New research has found that one of the main underlying causes of most allergies is a lack of probiotics in the intestines. When levels are low, toxins are allowed to re-enter the blood stream, causing the immune system to focus on eradicating these invasive compounds rather than destroying the allergic substances. [40]

* * *

Well, that not only ends the chapter on probiotics and your good gut bacteria, it also ends the part of the book that has dealt with the

90 essential nutrients, along with which foods and supplements are best to obtain them from.

Hopefully, the information that has been presented to you so far has outright convinced you of why your body ***must*** receive these nutrients every day... at all costs.

Consuming foods such as wheat grass, colloidal minerals, evening primrose oil, and a good quality probiotic supplement every day are guaranteed to protect us from any unwanted ailments and "diseases of civilization" (cancer, heart disease, diabetes, arthritis, etc).

I wouldn't say they make us bullet proof... but they sure go close!

* * *

In the next chapter entitled *Foods to avoid – foods to eat*, we'll be discussing the importance of making correct food choices and the direct impact this has on our health and well-being.

We'll also discuss which particular foods we need to be eating more of and which foods we need to be eating less of - or completely avoiding altogether.

Even though the foods and supplements I've talked about so far will keep us healthy, that doesn't give us free rein to go out and eat whatever we like.

It's essential that we still eat well and supply our body with foods that will enhance it – not harm it.

The incredible reward of looking good and feeling great really does make this a very worthwhile practice!

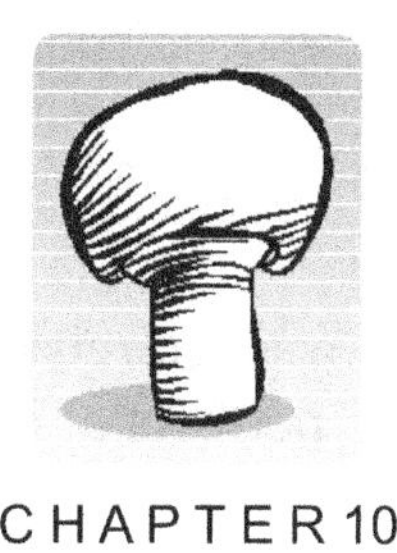

Foods to Avoid, Foods to Eat...

If you've been involved in the computer industry for any length of time you would have heard the old saying... "garbage in - garbage out".

What exactly does this mean?

Well, a computer will only give out the information that's first put into it by the user. So, if you put the wrong information in, you'll get the wrong information coming back out.

The funny thing is... our bodies work *exactly* the same!

If you put the wrong foods into your body, you'll get the same coming out performance-wise and health-wise (as you sow so shall you reap).

It's amazing how many people feed their body junk and garbage day after day and still expect it to perform at its peak and never break down.

It's just not going to happen Princess!

Think about this; if you had a prized racehorse, would you feed it junk food and let it lounge around watching TV all day?

Of course, you wouldn't!

You would make sure it was exercising and receiving the best nutrition possible in order to perform at its best.

Well, let me tell you something... *you're far more valuable than any racehorse!*

You owe it to yourself to get your body strong and healthy - that way, it will not only perform at its peak, it will also last its full amount of years without breaking down.

Who Cares About Nutrition?... Taste is all That Matters!

The problem with our eating habits today is we've been conditioned to believe that "taste is everything."

Most of us are more concerned with the food we eat satisfying our taste buds rather than how nutritious it is. I believe this is what's causing so many health problems today. And because people want their food to taste good, they'll usually cook with or add heaps of fat, sugar, processed salt, or other harmful ingredients, in order to achieve the taste they want.

I'm not saying that food shouldn't taste good either. What I am saying is that getting the balance right between taste AND nutritional value is what's important.

The other sad fact is food companies and food manufacturers know all too well how important taste is to us, so they fill their products with artificial colours, flavours, enhancers, sugar, processed salt, raising agents, and numerous other chemicals - all of which are designed to make the foods we eat taste better and be more appealing. Even our fruits and vegetables contain various dyes and waxes so their pigment appears darker and they "shine" more.

Unfortunately, this practice has now provided us with foods that are virtually devoid of any nutrition and are actually harmful instead of healthy.

I remember a prominent veterinarian once saying that if you want your family pets to live as long as possible, **never** feed them human food!

That certainly tells you something doesn't it?

A Society of Fast Food Junkies

If we look at today's thriving take away and fast food industry, we have to ask ourselves just why and how has this industry grown and become so popular so quickly?

I believe there are two basic reasons...

The first; because people today lead such busy lifestyles, they don't have time to prepare decent "home-made" meals anymore (or they can't be bothered), so it's much easier to grab a "bite to eat" from a take away store or fast food drive through.

The second and main reason is because fast food tastes pretty good!

I'll be the first to agree with this.

The downside is fast food is nothing but crap - and that's putting it politely! It has next to no nutritional value and contains toxic substances that are detrimental (deadly) to our health.

Here's just a short list of some of the most common ingredients found in take away and fast foods (that we know about) ...

- Rancid fats and heterocyclic amines

- Trans-fatty acids

- Acrylamides

- Sodium nitrite/nitrate

- Propylene glycol

- Silicon dioxide

- Ammonium sulphate

- TBHQ (a type of butane)

- Dimetylpolysiloxane (silly putty!)

- Azodicarbonamide (used to make rubber yoga mats)

- Food dyes

- Synthetic cysteine (made from duck feathers and human hair)

- Carminic acid (beetle extract)

- Cellulose (wood pulp)

- Mechanically separated meat (more commonly known as "pink slime")

- GMO's

- MSG

- Cancer causing phthalates

In addition, health experts now believe the terrible obesity epidemic we're experiencing today is primarily caused by the over-consumption of fast food and junk food.

So, if you like the idea of consuming known carcinogens, or human hair and duck feathers (yum), or even a bit of silly putty, then go right ahead and eat that horrible garbage posing as food. But keep this in mind... if it doesn't come back to bite you in the ass right now, it most certainly will further down the track!

The Danger of Refined Sugars and Soft Drinks

Refined sugars and soft drinks definitely fit into the junk food category and are of no benefit to us health-wise.

The amount of simple sugars and soft drinks that are consumed by people today is a real cause for concern. This unhealthy dietary practice has now left us with an "immune-deficient," "weak-boned" society – the likes of which have never been seen before.

The main problem with the consumption of refined sugars and soft drinks *is they extract valuable calcium from the bones.* This is another reason (along with a lack of calcium, magnesium, boron and vitamin D) why conditions such as osteoporosis, arthritis, kidney stones, back problems, loose teeth and tooth decay are so prevalent today. According to the *Harvard Medical Nurses' Health Study*, drinking carbonated drinks can actually increase some of these conditions in an individual by a whopping 500%! Research has also shown that diabetes, heart disease and cancer are closely linked to the over-consumption of refined sugars and soft drinks. [19,12]

When it comes to soft drinks, not only are they full of sugar, they also contain a substance called phosphoric acid. Phosphoric acid wreaks havoc on the bones and virtually sucks them dry of calcium, magnesium and boron. Once these three key minerals are leached from the bones, bone density is lowered severely – to the point where even a minor fall can cause a devastating fracture or breakage.[19]

Researchers now believe the consumption of soft drinks by women, especially pregnant women, is one of the reasons why many babies are now being born with soft, porous bones. Of course, a calcium, magnesium, boron and vitamin D deficiency is the other major cause. [19]

We also find young children and teenagers consuming soft drinks more than ever. It comes as no surprise that softened brittle bones and diseases such as arthritis - which were once diseases only seen in the elderly - are now affecting our younger generation.

In addition to this, phosphoric acid, along with carbon dioxide, not only give soft drinks their "fizz," they also burn your insides out! [12]

Diet Drinks are Even Worse...

Now don't think that diet soft drinks and diet sodas are any better for you – because these are actually worse. Some of the artificial sweeteners used in these products (particularly aspartame) have been found to be extremely harmful – even deadly!

Overwhelming evidence has now been able to prove that the sweetener, aspartame (also known as NutraSweet, Equal, AminoSweet or artificial sweetener E951) can cause diseases such as multiple sclerosis, Alzheimer's disease, brain tumors, and lupus, along with birth defects, blindness, mental retardation, seizures, manic depression, panic attacks, and other neurological problems.[41,42]

Aspartame is especially dangerous to diabetics as it keeps the body's blood sugar at an uncontrollable level, causing many sufferers to collapse and go into a coma! [41,42]

The problem with aspartame is it attacks the entire nervous system, especially the neurons in the brain.

World-renowned expert on aspartame poisoning, Dr H.J. Roberts, explains in his book, *Defence Against Alzheimer's Disease,* how aspartame is escalating Alzheimer's to a level of serious concern. Thirty-year-old women are now being diagnosed with this debilitating disease (most diet drinks and other diet products are consumed by women). Dr Roberts has also stated that: *"Consuming aspartame at the time of conception can cause birth defects."* [41,42]

At a world conference of the American College of Physicians, it was stated (regarding aspartame): *"We are talking about a plague of neurological diseases caused by this deadly poison."* [41,42]

What's interesting about aspartame is it's found in nearly all diet and "sugar free" products, yet it's not even a diet product. In fact, according to the Congressional Record... *"It makes you crave carbohydrates and will make you FAT"*. [41,42]

How ridiculous is that?

Aspartame is not a natural substance either - far from it in fact. It's a synthetic chemical made up of three key ingredients; aspartic acid, phenylalanine and methanol. Aspartame is made by the cultivation and growth of genetically modified E. coli bacteria, which defecate (poop, in laymen's terms) the proteins that contain the aspartic acid-phenylalanine amino acid segment. This is what is then used to make "aspartame." [41,42]

Nice right?

I really love the way they give it a name like "NutraSweet" or "AminoSweet." Sounds healthy, doesn't it? Instead, it's an extremely harmful and deadly poison that's currently wreaking havoc on the innocent and unsuspecting human population!

If you suffer from memory loss, headaches, mood swings, vertigo, dizziness, depression, blurred vision, anxiety attacks, spasms, cramps, shooting pains, numbness in your legs, joint pain, tinnitus, slurred speech, or have fibromyalgia symptoms - and you consume diet sodas or other diet products - then you could very well have "aspartame poisoning." [41,42]

Any product that contains artificial sweetener 951, NutraSweet, Equal, Spoonful, Neotame, or AminoSweet, should be avoided at all costs.

For more information on aspartame, I recommend you visit Dr Joseph Mercola's website (mercola.com) and take the time to read and watch some of his powerful articles and videos on this incredibly dangerous substance.

So What About Dairy Foods? Are They Healthy?

Milk in its natural state (i.e., straight from the cow) is a food rich in vitamins, minerals, amino acids, live enzymes and fat. The problem is though, most of us don't have access to "real milk."

The milk we buy from the supermarket is pasteurized and homogenized. When milk is pasteurized during the processing stage, it's exposed to high temperatures (130-170°F). As a result, most of the valuable nutrients are killed off, along with crucial live enzymes. This leaves the milk with very little nutritional value.

Homogenization is the process in which the cream from the milk is broken down and dissolved instead of being left to float at the top. Homogenized milk is very difficult for the body to digest and causes plaque and contamination in the lower intestine.

All processed milk is nothing but "dead milk" - even if it is low fat or fortified with extra iron or calcium. Interestingly, an experiment was done where a large number of calves were fed pasteurized/homogenized milk instead of normal cow's milk.

They all died from it!

The other downside with milk is the calcium it contains (which is the reason most people drink it) has such a coarse texture that absorbability is extremely poor. Remember I said earlier that Australia, New Zealand and the United States consume more milk per capita than any other countries in the world, yet still have the highest rates of osteoporosis? This is why. [3]

The bottom line with milk and other dairy products is this...

If you're one of the few people who has access to milk straight from a cow then go ahead and drink it.

If you're like most of us though and can only buy processed milk then don't be looking to gain any nutritional value from it.

And whatever dairy foods you eat or drink, forget about consuming them for your daily supply of calcium. It's a pointless exercise!

The Meat Controversy... To Eat or Not to Eat?

There's been a strong debate raging for many years as to which is healthier – a vegetarian diet or an omnivorous (eating all kinds of foods) diet.

Many vegetarians argue that man isn't meant to eat meat because biologically, he belongs in the same class as the anthropoid apes (they, like man, have flat teeth, flat nails and long convoluting intestines). These animals are strictly frugivorous.

Meat eating animals, on the other hand (lion, tiger, dog, wolf, etc), have sharp teeth, strong claws and short intestines in which to kill, eat and digest their prey.

The vegetarian argument is that if humans were meant to eat meat, we would have been given the physical equipment and internal organs, the same as flesh eating animals? In other words, we would have been designed both internally and externally to consume meat.

Now, I certainly don't disagree with what they're saying, however, in regards to human health and longevity, there's still no convincing evidence that proves being a vegetarian contributes to a person living longer.

There was an interesting article in the May edition of *The Denver Post* back in 1996 on a study that involved all of the people who were over the age of a hundred and living in the state of Colorado at the time (the oldest was 111 years of age).

415 centenarians took part in the State Social Services study and the idea was to interview each person to try and establish if there was one "overwhelming factor" that contributed to their longevity.

Each one of the participants was subjected to five pages of intensive questions and the overall data was then analysed.

What researchers found was there were both men and women in the group and every type of religion, race and culture were present. So there was no overwhelming factor in that sense.

Interestingly, after all of the extensive questions that each of the participants were asked, there was only *one* factor that was 100% universal with all four hundred and fifteen people. Every one of them were meat eaters and ate meat at least twice a day. There was not one vegetarian in the group! [19]

So you have to ask the question? If meat is so bad for us then why aren't these people all dead? [3]

Now, in defence of the vegans and vegetarians, there have also been plenty who have lived over the age of 100 as well. Here's just a few...

Loreen Dinwiddie – 108 year old vegan

Angeline Strandal – 104 year old vegetarian

Beatrice Wood – 105 year old vegetarian (this was the woman whom the movie TITANIC was based on).

Blanche Mannix – 105 year old vegetarian

Catherine Hagel - 114 year old vegetarian

Charles "Hap" Fisher – 102 year old vegetarian

Christian Mortensen – 115 year old vegetarian (oldest documented living man)

Gladys Stanfield – 105 year old lifelong vegetarian

Fauja Singh – 100 year old vegetarian

Florence Ready – 101 year old raw food vegetarian

Personally, I believe that whether you eat meat or you don't is not anywhere near as important *as making sure you take in all of the essential nutrients every day!*

The problem I see with being a vegetarian or vegan in today's world (and not taking nutritional supplements) is because of the lack of nutrients contained in our fruits, vegetables and grains, these people can end up becoming more severely deficient than the omnivores.

Unfortunately, vegetarians are at a distinct disadvantage compared to meat eaters.

Why is this?

At least there are still good amounts of nutrients contained in meats such as beef, chicken and fish. In our fruits, vegetables and grain produce, there's barely any!

Man Screws up Again...

Needless to say, when it comes to meat, you do need to be very careful where you purchase your supply from. Just as man has contaminated our fruits, vegetables and grains with artificial chemicals and pesticides, he's also contaminated our meat products with growth stimulants, hormones, antibiotics, steroids and other chemicals (hence why young boys are now growing man boobs). Even certain fish and other marine life have been found to be suspect as a result of the pollution in our waters.

When it comes to eating meat, the most important part is actually how you cook it. Overcooking, burning and char-grilling meat is extremely toxic and dangerous.

If we go back to the *Harvard Medical School Nurses' Health Study* (121,000 nurses studied for 20 years) they found that eating burnt animal fat from overcooked meat increases your risk of breast, colorectal and prostate cancers dramatically.[19]

And in November 1998, The University of South Carolina published the results of a large study on meat and they found that if you cook your meat well-done you *increase* your rate of breast and prostate cancers by 462%. [19]

This is where the mistaken belief came from that eating meat cause's cancer. It's not the meat at all – it's how it's cooked.

So if you're a meat eater... never overcook or char-grill your meat!

Meat has also received a bad rap in the past because studies have shown that eating too much can raise cholesterol levels.

What's important to keep in mind though is that *the body actually needs cholesterol* the same as it needs Vitamin C or calcium. The problem is excess cholesterol in the blood.

The human body can only make 10% of its daily cholesterol need - the remaining 90% must come from the foods we eat. People have become so paranoid these days about cholesterol and cutting out all fats from their diet that many are now cholesterol deficient. [1]

For example, the human brain by weight is 75% pure cholesterol. And the protective layer surrounding your brain (myelin) is almost 100% pure cholesterol. If you get really good at cutting out all meat, eggs, and other cholesterol containing foods from your diet then you'll find in about 10 to 12 years this insulating material around your brain will be gone, your brain will no longer function properly (it needs this "insulation" for the electrical signals to work), and you'll probably end up with dementia or Alzheimer's disease! [1,19]

So in conclusion to the whole "meat controversy" debate – it seems that meat is not as bad for us as what we've been led to believe. If it is then why aren't all of the people who enjoy longevity vegetarians?

Oh, and in case you're wondering, I'm actually a vegetarian myself (switched 5 years ago). I did this purely for moral and ethical reasons, not for health reasons.

What About Eggs? Are They Okay?

While we're on the subject of cholesterol, let's have a look at another food we've been told to avoid because of the amount of cholesterol it contains – the good old fashioned chook egg.

This food would have to be one of nature's true masterpieces. It

contains all of the essential nutrients and nourishment an unborn
chick requires to reach maturity.

For humans, eggs are considered to be a "perfect" protein and
nutrient source. They contain high amounts of amino acids,
vitamins, minerals, antioxidants, and yes, fat and cholesterol.

But you may well ask, aren't we supposed to avoid eating eggs
because of the cholesterol they contain? Well thankfully sanity has
prevailed on this one, mainly due to the results of a study by the
American Heart Association...

In this study, they took 141 healthy people with an average
cholesterol reading of 227 (the normal range at the time of the study
was 220-270). For six months these people were required to eat two
eggs for breakfast every morning. After the six-month period was
up their cholesterol levels were re-tested.

What researchers found was the groups average cholesterol levels
did in fact go up after the 6 months – but they only went up by a
minuscule 6 points. [19]

In response, here's what the American Heart Association came
out and said at their annual meeting on November 15th, 1995: *"We
always assumed that eggs were bad for you because they contained
cholesterol, but it now appears after this simple study that two eggs
a day won't hurt."* [19]

And in the *New England Journal of Medicine* there was an article
titled "Normal Cholesterol in 88 Year Old Man Eating 25 Eggs a
Day." [19]

This fella, nicknamed the egg man, had been eating an astonishing
25 eggs every day for over 15 years, and yet his cholesterol levels
were perfectly normal!

So don't be afraid to eat your two eggs for breakfast. They're an important source of quality nutrients and other essential growth factors.

Organic Free Range Only...

When it comes to purchasing your eggs, *never* buy any that come from battery fed and housed chickens (commercially raised). These eggs are full of antibiotics, chemicals and synthetic colourings (for instance, certain colourings such as Xanthophylls are added to their feed so the yolk appears a rich, "healthy" looking orange colour instead of the pale orange that comes from organic chicken eggs). [3]

These eggs are highly suspect and should not be eaten.

Only ever buy certified organic free-range eggs from a trusted supplier - or even better, raise your own chooks!

Butter vs Margarine – Which One is Really Better?

This is another one that's had most of us confused for years.

One minute we're being told that butter is healthier, then margarine, then butter, and now we're back to margarine again!

So which is the better of the two?

Well, butter is not only the better choice, it's the *only* choice in my view.

Margarine is made from commercially processed "hydrogenated" vegetable oils and contains deadly trans-fatty acids. Even if they display the "trans fat free" or "no trans fat" label, these margarines still contain a certain amount of trans fatty acids (they can't get rid of them completely), along with hexane and other industrial chemicals. But worse than this is the fact that most of the refined vegetable oils used for making margarine are actually "oxidized" rancid oils. This is something margarine manufactures definitely don't want you to know about.

Some manufacturers even claim their margarine contains healthy essential fatty acids. This is totally misleading as commercial oils and refined vegetable oils are devoid of any EFAs due to the extreme heat they are subjected to during processing.

The bottom line here is margarine is an unnatural, man-made product that should be avoided at all costs. Commercially produced butter is not totally natural either (the milk used is usually pasteurized milk). However, it's still a healthier option than margarine by a country mile – especially if you go with grass-fed butter made with raw milk. As an alternative, you can try vegan butter, which actually tastes pretty good!

And the Cholesterol Factor?

Of course, some nutritionists argue that being an animal fat, butter is high in cholesterol (yes, we're back to this cholesterol thing again). It's interesting to note, however, that statistics show in the major butter-producing countries like Sweden and Denmark, where their consumption is high, they actually have more normal cholesterol levels and less heart disease than many of the countries that avoid butter. [3]

This is another example of why a dietary imbalance of too many refined/processed foods and a lack of the essential nutrients contributes more to excessive cholesterol than eating so-called "high cholesterol foods" such as butter and eggs. And besides, it's estimated that only around 20% of your blood cholesterol comes from your diet anyway!

Chocoholics, Beware of the Fine Print!

Chocolate is indeed one of those foods that just about *everybody* enjoys eating. I'd say it would probably be the most popular "sweet" in the world today. But is it really healthy?

Well, yes and no.

No all chocolates are created equal, so whether chocolate is actually good or bad for you depends greatly on the type of chocolate and the ingredients used. The main ingredient in most chocolate is cocoa, however, cacao is now being used in many of the "healthier" chocolate alternatives.

Both come from the cocoa pod.

The difference between the two is cocoa gets heated to high temperatures during the extraction process, whereas, raw cacao is extracted via the more beneficial, cold-pressed method. Both cocoa and cacao contain some very powerful, naturally-occurring antioxidants including resveratrol and catechins, along with many of the essential nutrients. Because cacao is still in its natural, raw state, it's definitely the healthier option of the two.

Dark chocolate contains the highest amount of cacao and cocoa (the darker the chocolate the higher the content). This is the only type of chocolate you should eat. Not surprisingly, commercially processed chocolate contains loads of added sugar and artificial additives so definitely <u>do not</u> eat this rubbish! Only buy organic, fair trade dark chocolate that contains at least 70% cacao.

Dark chocolate can also taste quite bitter so rather than sugar being used to sweeten, make sure you find a brand that uses the healthier alternatives – stevia or monk fruit. Or instead of buying your chocolate (and paying a hefty price for it) go out and purchase some organic cacao powder and make your own chocolate treats instead.

Here's some of the health benefits of eating a little raw, dark chocolate every day...

- Improves blood flow (anti-thrombotic), lowers blood pressure

- Lowers bad cholesterol and raises good cholesterol

- Lowers your risk of cardiovascular disease

- Protects against UV damage and improves skin condition

- Improves brain function and has neuroprotective benefits

- Lowers insulin resistance, making it healthy for diabetics

- Helps prevent cancer

- Contains anti-inflammatory properties

- Reduces stress hormone production

- Improves healthy gut bacteria

Tea or Coffee Anyone?...

To say these two refreshments are popular would be a gross understatement. Apart from water, tea and coffee are *the* most consumed beverages world-wide.

Many people, including myself, simply cannot start their day without a hot cup of Joe or pot of tea. Both tea and coffee (more so tea) have been consumed for thousands of years and their beneficial effects are well documented. Thankfully, the research findings that continue to show up on the health benefits of tea and coffee keep getting better and better!

Tea and coffee contain some of the most potent antioxidants of any food or drink, along with many of the vital nutrients we need. They also contain caffeine, which is actually beneficial in moderate amounts - not detrimental as was once thought.

The main antioxidants in tea and coffee are substances called polyphenols, however, coffee also contains chlorogenic acid and tea, particularly green tea, contains the very powerful catechin antioxidants. Organic Matcha green tea contains the highest amount of antioxidants (by a long shot), so if you can find some Matcha, this should definitely be your first choice.

Drinking anywhere from 3-5 cups a day of either tea or coffee is beneficial according to the latest findings. In the 2015 edition of *Dietary Guidelines for Americans*, a government advisory committee stated that up to 5 cups of coffee a day could be consumed with no detrimental effects. With tea, there's no set recommendation or amount that should be consumed each day - so you can essentially go ahead and drink as much as you like. Most studies done on tea consumption have found that the more tea you drink the more benefits you receive!

Here's some of the health benefits of regularly drinking tea and coffee...

- *They make you smarter and starve off neurodegenerative diseases such as Alzheimer's* - Controlled trials in humans have shown that both tea and coffee significantly improve brain function - particularly memory, mood, vigilance, energy levels, reaction times and general cognitive function. Studies have also shown that tea and coffee drinkers have up to a 65% lower risk of developing Alzheimer's disease and dementia than non drinkers. With Parkinson's disease it's up to a 60% reduction.

- *Tea and coffee improve physical performance and help burn body fat* – Caffeine increases the levels of the "fight or flight" hormone epinephrine (adrenaline) in the blood, along with causing fat cells to break down body fat to use as energy. Caffeine can boost your physical performance by 11-12% on average and increase your metabolic rate (fat burning capacity) anywhere from 3-11%.

- *They lower your risk of type II diabetes* – Over 300 million people world-wide have type II diabetes. Studies show that people who drink the most tea and coffee have a 23-50% - and even up to 67% - lower risk of developing this disease than non drinkers. The polyphenols in green tea and coffee also help to regulate glucose in the body, so these beverages can benefit someone who is already type II diabetic. In one study they found diabetics who drank tea or coffee had a 30% reduced risk of death compared to diabetics who avoided these drinks.

- *Tea and coffee are good for your heart* – It was once thought that caffeine increased systolic blood pressure, but the longer-term studies haven't found any connection. Although caffeine can initially cause a small rise in blood pressure (3-4 mm/Hg), this goes away once you begin drinking tea or coffee regularly. Tea and coffee have actually been found to reduce your risk of stroke by 20% and reduce your risk of heart attack by one fifth according to a large study performed by the *University Medical Center Utrecht Netherlands*. Tea consumers were the big winners in the study as they managed to reduce their risk of developing heart disease by 36% compared to 20% with coffee drinkers.

- *They lower your risk of developing cancer* – Tea and coffee are particularly protective against two types of cancers,

Colorectal cancer (15% lower risk and 52% reduced risk of reoccurrence if you already have the disease) and liver cancer (40% lower risk). Tea and coffee have also been found to reduce the risk of oral cancer by 39%, prostate cancer by 60%, brain cancer by 40%, breast cancer by 49%, and endometrial cancer by 19%, along with significantly reducing the risk of melanoma skin cancers.

- *Tea and coffee fight depression and make you happier* – Depression is a serious disorder. Globally, an estimated 350 million people suffer from this affliction. Thankfully, tea and coffee have been shown to help... In a Harvard Medical study published back in 2011, women who drank 4 or more cups a day of tea or coffee had a 20% lower risk of becoming depressed. Another study involving 208,424 individuals found that those who drank 4 or more cups each day were 53% less likely to want to try and commit suicide.

- *They help you live longer* – Research published in the *New England Journal of Medicine* revealed that tea and coffee consumption significantly reduce your overall risk of premature death. And the interesting part is they found that the more you drink the more you lower your risk! In two other large studies, regular consumption of tea and coffee were associated with a 20% reduced risk of premature death in men and a 26% reduced risk of premature death in women. [51]

For me personally, I much prefer tea over coffee, especially during the warmer months. Tea is incredibly refreshing and you still get the same benefits as what you do with coffee (particularly the caffeine boost). Tea also keeps you going for longer as it gives you a more slower energy release, whereas coffee gives you that quick hit that can fade just as fast. The other down side to coffee is it's a strong diuretic and drinking it regularly makes you pee all the time!

To finish off, I'll leave you with an interesting piece of trivia about the Japanese and green tea...

When you look at all of the industrialized countries in the world, the Japanese have the longest life span. They also have 85% less cancer than Americans and 85% less cardio vascular disease, yet they consume twice as much salt per day, three times as much fat and cholesterol, and are the heaviest smokers in the world! [19]

What's their secret?

They all drink at least 4-6 cups of green tea, particularly Matcha green tea, everyday!

Other Foods We Need to Avoid....

It's now an established fact that the over-consumption of refined and processed foods is one of the major causes of disease and ill health in the Western world today (of course, a lack of the essential nutrients is another). [3]

These foods are nothing but "dead foods" and provide absolutely zero nourishment. Instead, they harm and overburden the body by giving it an unnecessary (and extra) workload to perform.

Remember this important maxim... *Any food that has been heated, treated or altered from its natural state is not going to contribute to good health!*

Aside from the refined/processed foods already discussed, other unhealthy foods we need to avoid include; any refined or processed food that contains high fructose corn syrup (HFCS), along with refined sugar and flour products such as pies, pastries, biscuits, cakes, commercial lollies, jams, ice cream, nutrition/muesli bars, sweetened fruit juices, chewing gum, jellies, and canned fruits with sugar syrup.

In addition to these, all other refined, processed, preserved, artificially coloured or flavoured and chemically treated foods need to be avoided. These include; canned foods, spaghetti and macaroni (except wholemeal), potato crisps, white polished rice, packaged desserts, junk food and fried foods.

Processed breakfast cereals such as Rice Bubbles, Rice Krispies, Cornflakes, Puffed Wheat, Fruit Loops, etc., are also nutrient-dead foods and contain about as much nutrition as the cardboard boxes they're packed in!

Tip: If you want to check what the main ingredients are in any processed food they are listed on the side of the item from highest amount to least amount. For instance, if the first ingredient is sugar, then sugar is what that processed food is primarily made up of. If the last ingredient is a preservative, then this makes up the smallest component of the food.

Healthy Foods We Need to Eat...

The foods we need to be eating every day to stay healthy are the tried-and-true staples. The most important ones, as you've probably already guessed, are fruits and vegetables – along with herbs and spices. Actually, the vast majority of your diet should consist of fresh, raw, organically grown (if possible) fruits, vegetables, spices and herbs. We can never feed our bodies too much of these powerhouse foods.

As I've said repeatedly, eating a diet high in fruit and vegetables (especially green leafy vegetables) greatly reduces our risk of developing a wide range of diseases including cancer and heart disease. Many herbs and spices such as tumeric, ginger, cinnamon and cayenne pepper have also been recognized for their anti-cancer and heart protecting properties. These foods not only supply us with vital nutrients in their pure and natural form, they also supply us with some of nature's hidden nutritional benefits as well.

Be Careful Where You Get Your Produce From

Certainly, one of the most important issues today regarding fruits, vegetables, and herbs and spices, is where to purchase them from.

Because of the way these are commercially grown (i.e., mineral deficient soils, the use of herbicides, pesticides, GMO's, artificial dyes, waxes, etc.) it's essential, where possible, that the produce we buy is organically grown and non GMO.

There are now many retailers that stock only certified organically grown, biodynamically grown and non GMO food and produce. If you're unable to find one then your local health food store may be able to help - or instead, you can always find an organic food retailer online.

Also consider that there are different interpretations of what "organically grown" produce is. Just because something is said to be grown organically, doesn't necessarily mean it's grown in mineral rich soils. It can just mean it's grown without the use of pesticides and chemicals, so be sure to find out. Look for the "100% Certified Organic" stamp as well to make sure they're non-GMO.

Evidently, a far better (and cheaper) alternative to buying organically grown fruits, vegetables and herbs is to grow your own. There are plenty of books available on organic gardening to help you out. It's not hard to do, and at least by growing your own food you know exactly what it contains and what you're eating.

Furthermore, you can now purchase specific mineral fertilizers that contain the full spectrum of minerals to replace back into the soil. This means you can grow your own "mineral rich" herbs, fruits and vegetables without the use of pesticides... and save yourself heaps of money in the process!

The Next Type of Foods...

After fruits, vegetables, herbs and spices, the next type of foods we should be including in our diet are legumes, whole grains, seeds and nuts.

These foods should also be in their natural state (unprocessed) and eaten either raw or after a minimal amount of cooking or boiling.

Legumes are incredibly rich in essential nutrients, healthy fibers and carbohydrates. They're also a great source of easily digestible (and high quality) protein.

Whole grains such as black rice, whole oats, millet and buckwheat are packed with valuable carbohydrates for energy and soluble fibre for a healthy colon. Wheat is also a whole grain but does contain gluten, so be aware of this (wheatgrass is free of gluten though).

Seeds such as linseeds (flaxseeds), sunflower and pumpkin seeds contain fiber, essential fatty acids, and many of the essential nutrients, while fermented soya beans (technically legumes) contain protein, EFA's, probiotics and isoflavones.

In regards to isoflavones, studies have found that these compounds benefit women suffering with menopause and PMS as they are similar in structure to human oestrogen – so they help the body maintain normal levels of this crucial hormone. In addition to this, isoflavones also protect against heart disease and cancer, including prostate, breast, colon, rectum, stomach and lung cancers. Just remember to eat fermented soya beans (Natto) as this is much more beneficial than regular soy.

The Final Type of Foods...

The last type of foods we can consume are meats. Eggs can be included in this category as well.

The benefit of meat is it's high in protein and is also a good source of vitamins and minerals, and yes - fat. Likewise, eggs contain a high amount of quality protein, along with many of the other essential nutrients, including fat and cholesterol.

These foods can be eaten everyday if desired, but should only make up about 20% of your total daily diet/calorie intake.

If you're vegetarian or vegan then simply include more fruits, vegetables, herbs, legumes, whole grains, nuts and seeds in your diet.

Note: When it comes to eating meat, this DOES NOT include any processed meats such as sausages, salami, fish fingers, fried chicken, etc. These fit into the same category as other processed foods and should not be eaten. With red meat, be sure to eat lean red meat and try to avoid any fatty meat such as chops, schnitzels, etc.

The Big Deception – Why Many Consumers are Being Fooled and Ripped off!

Now that we've had a look at the foods we need to avoid and the foods we need to be eating, let's take a look at an issue that's rarely talked about by the mainstream media, but one that I feel is important and needs to be brought to people's attention.

It concerns the blatant use of misleading advertising by food companies and manufactures in order to sell their products. Most people aren't even aware that this is happening. But unfortunately, it is, and many consumers are being sucked in and ripped off "big time" by purchasing what they think are healthier foods (and paying more for them in most cases), but instead, are getting a rubbish product that you wouldn't even give to your dog if you knew what was really in it!

Profits Before People

There's no doubt that we as a society are more health-conscious today than what we were fifteen to twenty years ago.

We're continually hearing about the importance of receiving enough calcium, magnesium, iron, folate, Vitamin C, fiber, etc., from our diets, along with other things such as keeping our cholesterol level down, avoiding cancer, heart disease, diabetes, and so on.

It's certainly obvious that people are now looking to buy healthier foods and are looking for healthier choices. It's become a real demand. The problem with this is food companies and manufacturers are aware of this and are trying to cash in on the demand by supplying foods that are supposed to be healthier for us, but in actual fact are no different – and in many cases are even worse.

A prime example of this is the adding of synthetic vitamins and minerals to foods such as cereals, breads, spreads, milk, and so forth. The type of vitamins and minerals used in these products are cheaply sourced synthetic versions that the body cannot absorb. Of course, these products are then heavily promoted as being high in iron or calcium or folate, etc., so you'll go out and buy them.

Do not fall for this despicable advertising!

Remember this, corporate companies are only concerned with profits and their bottom line. So, if it means having to deceive you, the unwary customer, in order to hit their profit targets then that's what they'll do.

The only way you're going to receive the nutrients you need every day is through the consumption of natural foods - not processed foods that have had a few cheap vitamins and minerals thrown in!

Other marketing scams to watch out for include:

• Bold labelling printed on processed foods describing them as "low in fat," "98% fat free," "cholesterol free," and so forth - but which are actually higher in fat than other similar products.

• Foods being promoted as "all natural" or "natural ingredients" when they still contain refined sugars, preservatives, and artificial additives.

• Margarines being promoted as good sources of essential fatty acids, when in reality they contain next to none (but do contain lots of toxic fats).

• Many commercial yogurts sold in supermarkets are supposed to contain high amounts of acidophilus and bifidus cultures. Instead, they contain high amounts of sugar and artificial additives. [18]

• Most so-called sports drinks and energy drinks on the market are nothing but sugar drinks and won't "hydrate" you any quicker than drinking good old fashioned water.

• Personal care products (shampoos, conditioners, soaps, skin care products, etc.) being advertized as "natural" when they still contain harmful chemicals such as sodium lauryl sulphate, propylene glycol, and others.

• Toothpastes that contain added calcium (as if teeth are able to "miraculously" absorb the calcium from toothpaste and become stronger. *Give me a break!*).

The list of marketing scams is almost endless.

Remember to *always* read what the ingredients are on any product you buy so you know exactly what you're getting.

Don't just buy a product because it's fortified with extra iron or calcium, or the label says "all natural ingredients," or it has "98% fat free" printed boldly on the label. Make sure you check it out for yourself. Most of these products are more expensive, yet provide no additional benefit.

…Now I know this is slightly off track, but have you also noticed that the products you buy from the supermarket are continuing to get smaller? Food companies have been guilty of this deceitful and sneaky practice for years. For instance, something that weighed 250 grams a few years ago might now only weigh 180 grams…. but it still costs the same!

It's definitely time for us to fight back, and going completely raw and natural so you don't need their products is certainly one way to do this.

Artificial Additives – Not as Harmless as we May Think…

Nearly all of the processed foods available on the market today contain artificial additives.

Even most of our natural produce contains artificial additives - and there seems to be no end to their use.

Consequently, the foods we are eating are a virtual chemical cocktail of dyes, waxes, fungicides, artificial colours, flavours, enhancers, bleaching agents, emulsifiers, preservatives, stabilisers, antioxidants… the list goes on.

What concerns me about the use of these chemicals and additives is that we're being told they pose no serious risk to our health.

This is certainly *not* the case, and if you take a look at the potential side effects of some of the artificial additives used in our foods today, you'll see what I mean:

High Fructose Corn Syrup (HFCS)

A cheap sweetener that's found in many refined and processed foods, particularly sodas and soft drinks, crackers, breakfast cereals, candy, yogurts, nutrition bars, and bread and baked goods. Studies show that HFCS causes weight gain, metabolic syndrome, type 2 diabetes, high triglyceride levels (a precursor to heart disease) and even premature death.

Sodium Nitrate/Nitrite

The International Agency for Research on Cancer (IARC) - a division of the World Health Organization (WHO) - recently came out and said that processed meats are now classified as "carcinogenic to humans." The reason? Processed meats contain nitrates and nitrites, both of which have been found to cause all sorts of serious health problems, particularly leukemia, brain tumors and colorectal cancer.

Caramel (150)

This artificial colouring is used to give certain foods and beverages their brown colour (e.g., cola drinks, chocolate, chocolate drink mixes, chocolate biscuits, various spreads, etc.). Most forms of this colouring are made with ammonia or sulphur dioxide. The safety level of this additive is highly suspect. It causes convulsions in animals and possible gastro-intestinal disorders in humans. It can also aggravate asthma and allergy problems in many people. [43]

Sulphites (220-228)

These are used in various foods and beverages including muesli bars and cordial. Sulphites are known to bring on asthma attacks in sufferers as the sulphur dioxide gas contained in them is a strong irritant to asthmatics. It's also recommended that sulphites be avoided by anyone with kidney and liver problems. [43]

Monosodium Glutamate (MSG)

MSG is used in a wide variety of foods as a flavor enhancer. It's known to be especially dangerous to certain people (asthmatics in particular) and can even kill! Small children and anyone sensitive to aspirin should also avoid this additive. Possible side effects include heart palpitations, headaches and nausea. [43]

Food Coloring's – Blue #1, Blue #2, Yellow #6 and Red #3

Found in products such as baked goods, candy and sodas. The Center for Science in the Public Interest revealed that all four of these food colorings contain dangerous cancer-causing properties.

Saccharin

Another toxic artificial sweetener that's been found to cause cancer, particularly ovarian cancer and cancer of the urinary tract.

So Why are These Additives Still in Our Foods Then?

Now you're probably wondering why any artificial additives that aren't natural are even allowed to be used in the foods we eat. If they have the potential to harm us in any way, shouldn't they be banned?

Well, here's the problem...

If these additives were to be banned then processed foods wouldn't keep as long, taste as good or look as good - and therefore the very powerful "big business" and multi national companies and corporations wouldn't make as much money and supply our all important governments with so much tax revenue! (So yes, it basically boils down to the fact that the almighty dollar is more important to these people than our health.)

But alas, it doesn't stop there.

Some food manufactures actually *fund* the very organizations that determine whether their products make the supermarket shelves - and then get to stay on the shelves or be taken off. [41,42]

As a result, these organizations are "bribed" into endorsing the manufacturers' products - which of course includes turning a blind eye to any harmful artificial additives they may contain - or risk losing their funding money.

In *The New York Times* there was an article by Marian Burros on how the American Dietetic Association (now called the Academy of Nutrition and Dietetics) receives money from the food industry in return for endorsing their products! [41,42]

How bad is this?

Remember I spoke earlier about the harmful effects of the artificial sweetener aspartame?

So why is this product still on the market then you may be wondering? Well, the company that created the product just happens to fund the Academy of Nutrition and Dietetics and the American Diabetes Association, and at one time also funded the Conference of the American College of Physicians annual meeting. [41,42]

With all of that funding money being given, who's going to say anything? (It's amazing, and to me, extremely sad just how many people will keep their mouths shut when there's money involved.)

A few years back an industry watchdog consulting group known as *Eat Drink Politics* published a terrific book titled *"And Now a Word From Our Sponsors,"* where it was revealed how the Academy of Nutrition and Dietetics (AND) accepts corporate sponsorships from many of the big name food companies, and has been doing so for a long time. Some of the big multi national food and beverage companies (whom I'm not going to name) have even been caught out paying nutrition experts to recommend their products as "healthy snacks."

And it seems the U.S. is not the only country caught up in this deceitful practice. The Dietitians Association of Australia recently came under fire for being in the pockets of some of the major food companies - accepting money and corporate sponsorships from these corporations as well. [49]

End Note...

So in conclusion to the use of artificial additives - just be aware that they're in most of the processed foods and personal care products on the market. Of course, some are harmful and some are less harmful. I've described only a few of the ones that can cause health problems.

For a complete description of all the artificial additives used in our foods and their possible side effects, you can purchase a handy little book entitled *Food Additives: A Shoppers Guide to What's Safe & What's Not* by Dr Christine H. Farlow, available from Amazon. This book is also valuable as it tells you the codes of most additives (manufacturers are not obliged to list the full names of any artificial additives they use and can instead just list their codes – for example, 950, 951, 220, and so forth).

Other Health Hazards That Kill...

I feel I cannot end this chapter without first discussing the health hazards of two of the biggest causes of poor health and early death in the world today – smoking and alcohol.

When it comes to smoking, you would have to be living on another planet not to know by now the dangers of this unhealthy practice. Cigarette smoking is responsible for more than 480,000 deaths each year in the United States, including nearly 42,000 deaths from second hand smoke exposure (passive smoking). We're talking about one in five deaths annually here, or 1,300 deaths every day!

The problem with cigarette smoke is it contains over eight different deadly poisons, including the heavy metal forms of arsenic, lead and cadmium. These poisons are difficult for the body to eliminate and so begin to build up until they eventually cause serious and irreparable damage.

Some of the health problems associated with cigarette smoking include anemia, high blood pressure (caused by blood vessel shrinkage), heart palpitations, vertigo and COPD, along with eventual heart disease and cancer - particularly lung cancer (still the biggest cancer killer in the U.S.). [3]

And don't think E-Cigarettes and vaping are any better either - they're actually worse! The chemicals produced from these devices have been found to be incredibly toxic to the heart and lungs (acetaldehyde, acrolein and formaldehyde are the 3 main chemicals). The FDA is yet to find **any** E-Cigarette safe, both for the user and for any unfortunate soul who breathes in that awful smelling (second hand) smoke. [50]

Alcohol, on the other hand, is a less talked about killer than cigarette smoking.

Most people don't believe that its continued use can cause health problems, yet many cases of liver disease and liver cancer (the fifth biggest cancer killer in the U.S.) can be traced back to the continued consumption of alcohol.

Aside from causing cirrhosis of the liver, alcohol can also cause heart complaints and irreversible brain damage. It depletes the body of many essential vitamins and minerals, including vitamin B and calcium. [3]

Additionally, alcohol contains a lot of empty calories, which means eating habits become disrupted and many regular drinkers find themselves gaining weight easily - men around the stomach (beer gut) and women around the hips and buttocks (wine glass look).

Research has actually shown that alcohol - minus the preservatives - *is* something that can be consumed safely, if it's in moderation (around one standard drink a day). Unfortunately, the average drinker doesn't know what moderation is.

Okay, there's my lecture on smoking and alcohol done. I feel better now!

* * *

That concludes this chapter on Foods to avoid – foods to eat.

Now that you know which foods to eat more of and which foods to eat less of, it's up to you to make the necessary effort to eat healthy.

If someone is frequently experiencing poor health, you usually only have to look at their diet to see why.

As I said at the beginning of this chapter, most people feed their body junk and garbage day after day and still expect it to perform at its peak and never break down.

It's just not going to happen!

You can't put square blocks into round holes.

In his book, *The Natural Way to Better Health and Longer Life,* Naturopath and health expert, Vaughan Bullivant, sums up with a bemusing quote what I've been saying:

> *"Having established the fundamental relationship between the food we eat and the efficient functioning of the cells of the body, why is it that the idea current in some circles today and shared by the general public is to the effect that it does not matter what we eat? It is taken for granted that the body in some miraculous way can transmute demineralised, devitalised foods into healthy tissues."* [3]

Indeed, this is the problem, and hopefully you no longer share in this belief, but now understand that what you feed and put into your body is absolutely vital for your overall health and crucial to your very survival!

* * *

In the next chapter entitled *Putting it all Together*, I have taken everything that has been discussed so far and outlined a simple, yet effective diet and supplementation plan. This plan not only supplies us with the vital 90 nutrients our bodies need every day, it also supplies us with foods that make the body perform strongly rather than the awful sluggishness that comes from eating nutrient dead, toxic foods.

Let's continue...

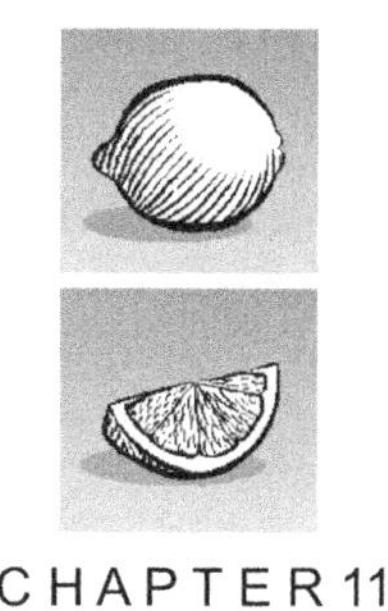

CHAPTER 11

Putting it all Together
The Ultimate Health and Longevity Program!

For us to fully benefit from the information that's been presented in this book, it's essential that we follow a simple diet and supplementation plan for optimum results.

Now I know the word "diet" can conjure up thoughts of having to starve yourself and go without all of your favourite foods forever.

Well, you can relax - this is not what I'm talking about.

This plan certainly does involve eating healthy foods, but it still allows you to enjoy a treat every now and then.

If you're overweight, you'll find yourself losing weight on this program. Likewise, if you're underweight, you'll find yourself gaining weight on this program as your metabolism stabilizes and helps your body naturally adjust to its ideal body weight. Your energy levels and overall sense of wellbeing will also increase dramatically, as will your resistance to illness and disease (not to mention your lifespan).

It really is a wonderful feeling when you know you're healthy on the inside and you look radiantly healthy on the outside as well!

Before Starting – What You Need to Know

There are a couple of things you need to keep in mind when starting this program.

The first, and probably the most important one is to begin *sloooowly!*

Sadly, I've seen so many people get all excited about eating healthy and go from a junk food addict to a health food addict in one day. A month or two later they're back to eating junk.

The sudden change, I'm guessing, was either too much for their body to handle or too much for their mind to handle (or both).

If, on the other hand, you begin a new diet program slowly, making small changes everyday, the body is better able to cope with these changes.

I believe that allowing yourself a "treat night" once a week makes it so much easier to eat healthy and stick to a healthy eating plan.

Most diets or healthy eating regimens don't allow you any real treats at all, so what usually happens is the eating plan is easy to follow for the first month or two while your enthusiasm is high, but it soon becomes more and more difficult (especially if you're suffering from pica).

You begin to crave ice cream, chocolate or some other type of junk food, and eventually, after you can stand it no longer, you "indulge" yourself. You then feel guilty and depressed because you've broken your diet. This makes you want to eat more, and because you've already broken your diet then "what the heck," you might as well eat more rubbish. Before you know it, your diet has gone out the window.

Studies clearly show that these types of super strict diets do not have very high long-term success rates.

With this program, it's easy to eat healthy all week because you know it will soon be your treat night (or cheat meal, or whatever you want to call it). Once it's gone, you're then satisfied and actually want to eat healthy again. You forget about eating any bad food and stick to your eating program easily. Then, before you know it, treat night has come around again!

I firmly believe that an eating plan must be realistic and workable. Remember, we aren't talking about a six-month diet or a twelve-month diet here. We're talking about a "rest of your life diet."

Don't Go Overboard and Stuff Yourself Stupid!

Now I know there are people out there who can eat healthy all of the time and never even want to eat any treats. If you're one of those people then that's great, I applaud you.

Unfortunately, I'm not one of them. I enjoy my treat night once a week!

And the thing is, eating one treat meal a week is not going to compromise your health either. Any more than that and it could be a different story. (Of course, you don't have to include this meal in your eating plan if you don't want to, but it's always there if you decide you want to have it).

What my wife and I do, for example, is instead of going out and buying takeaway pizza, we'll make our own using wholemeal pita bread, home-made tomato paste, pineapples, olives, mushrooms, egg plant, low fat cheese, etc. Or we'll make our own "healthier" (and better tasting) burgers and air-fried chips. That way, we still get to enjoy a treat without blowing the calorie budget!

If we happen to go out for dinner then we'll still eat somewhere that has good quality and reasonably healthy food (definitely no Chinese or Indian food) and still order something that's half decent from the menu - maybe even share a sweet after. Even a glass of wine or a beer (or two) if we feel like it as well.

Skip the Treat Meal if You're Unwell...

There is one final point that I do want to make in regards to having your treat meal for the week.

If you're allergic to food additives or are suffering from any type of ailment or disease then I would strongly suggest that you *don't* include this meal in your eating plan, at least for the time being.

The most important thing is your health and getting that up to 100%. Once you've done this, then you can begin to think about indulging yourself a little.

The Detoxing Phase Can Be a Little Uncomfortable

The second thing you need to keep in mind when you begin this program is that there is a cleansing process involved (a phenomenon known as Herxheimer's reaction).

Because we'll be consuming foods and supplements that cleanse the body of toxins, chemicals and other harmful substances, the first week or two for some people can be a little uncomfortable.

Depending on your age, you may have 30, 40, 50 years or more of toxins, chemicals and heavy metals built up in your body.

When you begin having foods that clean out these harmful substances, the body's eliminatory organs, such as the liver and kidneys, have to work harder until they can catch up and remove all of these toxins.

So be aware that you may suffer from a lack of energy, mild stomach upsets and excess bowel movements for the first week or two (most people usually only experience a slight loss of energy). Do remember though that this eliminatory process is perfectly normal and won't do you any harm.

And please, do not stop if you do experience any of these cleansing reactions. It's important that you continue on and push through the first couple of weeks. It really is well worth it, and I promise that once you do, you'll begin to feel better than you've felt in your entire life!

Also bear in mind that even after you've been on the program for a few months, your body may want to have one last clean out.

I've seen people become ill and even break out in a rash for a few days as the body has one last final cleansing. After a couple of days though, these people came back stronger and healthier than ever.

Keep in mind that it's going to take at least twelve months to reap the full health benefits of this program!

Like I said, your body may have had 30, 40, 50, or more years of toxic build up. Your immune system may also be very low or certain organs in your body, such as your liver and kidneys, may not be functioning at their optimum level. It's going to take time for the body to heal itself and become healthy. The important thing is to be patient.

Remember, Rome wasn't built in a day!

The Program...

So now that you know to begin slowly and what you may experience for the first couple of weeks and months of the program, let's go through it all step by step.

#1. The Fantastic Four – Wheat Grass Powder, Plant Based Colloidal Minerals, Probiotics and Evening Primrose Oil/Fish Oil

This is the most crucial part of our diet and supplementation plan as these foods and supplements are what will be supplying us with the 90 essential nutrients and other vital health factors we require for health and longevity.

When it comes to the wheat grass, it's important that it be consumed 10-20 minutes *before* food on an empty stomach. This allows for the maximum absorption and utilization of nutrients (the enzymes in the wheat grass also help with the digestion of your meal).

The liquid colloidal minerals can basically be consumed at any time, although either first thing in the morning or just before bedtime is considered the most beneficial.

With the probiotics, having them with the wheat grass is extremely important as the wheat grass is an excellent food source (prebiotic) for your good gut bacteria. This in turn makes the probiotics even more beneficial - by a large degree in fact.

The evening primrose oil and fish oil are also best consumed on an empty stomach and taken in divided doses. Having them with the other three is certainly okay but on their own will work even better.

So first thing in the morning we have our wheat grass powder, which can either be mixed with water or fruit juice (about half a glass of water should do it). You may prefer the fruit juice if you don't like the taste of the wheat grass, although you do eventually get used to it. I personally prefer mixing it with water because I really enjoy the taste!

With children, I've found that if you only use a small amount of water or juice with the wheat grass it's much easier for them to drink. And remember, wheat grass powder contains NO gluten, so it's completely safe for kids (and adults) who suffer from gluten sensitivity (celiac disease).

The important point to consider when starting out on the wheat grass is of course to begin slowly. This way you can usually avoid any cleansing reactions that may occur if the body begins to detox too quickly.

A half to one-teaspoon first thing in the morning for the first week should be okay. After that you can increase to one teaspoon in the morning and one teaspoon 20 minutes before your evening meal. Then a week or two later increase again to two teaspoons morning and night (total of four daily).

Alternatively, you could spread it out even more and have your wheat grass before each main meal. (It's far better to spread your wheat grass throughout the day rather than have it all in one drink.) Of course, with work commitments and so forth, it's not always viable or practical to be able to do this.

Children will benefit greatly from as little as one teaspoon daily and usually won't suffer any cleansing reactions. Adults can have anywhere from two up to eight or more teaspoons daily of wheat grass - depending on their nutritional requirements.

If your immune system is low or you're suffering from an illness or disease then you would benefit greatly from working up to having six to eight or more teaspoons daily.

After our wheat grass powder, we then need to have our colloidal mineral drink. This can either be consumed on its own (which is the preferred option) or you can pre-mix it in with your wheat grass (mixing both together does improve the taste of the wheat grass).

Exactly how much of the plant based colloidal minerals you need to have will depend on what brand you buy, but the rough rule of thumb is around 15 mls per 100 pounds (45 kilograms) of body weight.

Next on the agenda is our friendly lactobacillus bacteria. These are best obtained from lactobacillus (probiotic) supplements, which are usually available in either powdered or capsule form. You can also buy "kid friendly" probiotic supplements, which the little ones will love.

Two to three capsules or one to two teaspoons daily with your wheat grass will recolonize the gut with good bacteria and help maintain a healthy supply. With the children's formulas, one or two of the tablets or chewable gummies will give them everything they need.

Drinking kefir milk and kefir water, along with eating natural yogurt (or your own home made yogurt) and other powerful probiotic rich foods such as sauerkraut, kimchi, tempeh and home made pickles throughout the day will also provide an extra supply of friendly bacteria to the gut - so be sure to do this.

Finally, we have our evening primrose oil (EPO) and fish oil. Most of the EPO and fish oil supplements available on the market today are in capsule form, but there are some liquid versions which contain the pure oil.

With the EPO capsules (if they're 1000mg), around six of these daily or one to two teaspoons of the liquid evening primrose oil will do the trick. If you go with the fish oil (with the EPO), three to four

1000 mg capsules (or more) can be consumed daily. With children, one or two "fish oil gummies for kids" or one teaspoon of the liquid fish oil for kids is perfect.

Also make sure you have a tablespoon of the LSA mix I spoke about earlier in the chapter on essential fatty acids with one or two of your meals for an extra supply of EFA's.

Cost Effectiveness and Saving Money...

So there we have what I refer to as our "fantastic four" foods and supplements.

The beauty of these foods and supplements is they're not only extremely valuable to our health, they're also very cost effective.

I've read many health books and articles where they tell you you need to take a bunch of stuff like a multivitamin and mineral supplement, plus extra B-Vitamins, plus extra Vitamin C, plus Vitamin E, plus calcium, plus amino acids, plus ten different herbs, plus antioxidants, plus spirulina, plus this, plus that… and on and on it goes.

Now, all of this would cost an average family a small fortune every week and I doubt very much that most could afford it. With what I'm suggesting though, it's very affordable. Even more so if you purchase them at wholesale or close to wholesale prices (there are many supplement companies that are now doing this. Just search online).

If you also take a look at some of the extra treats and other nutritionally dead foods that usually go into your shopping trolley every week, you can see how either cutting down or eliminating these, and instead putting the money towards your wheat grass and other supplements, will help even more.

Of course, you could save money by only having the wheat grass and colloidal minerals every day (and still benefit tremendously just from these two). However, if you want to gain the full health benefits of this program then having all four is vital.

Also keep in mind that you cannot have too much of these foods and supplements.

Many people are scared to death that they will overdose on certain nutrients, particularly vitamins and minerals. While this can happen with some synthetic or inorganic vitamins and minerals, it CANNOT happen with nutrients that come from plant sources such as wheat grass and colloidal minerals.

These plant based sources are extremely safe!

The truth is… we actually need to be more concerned with *underdosing* rather than overdosing!!!

How Long Do I Need to Take These Supplements For?

This is a question I'm often asked.

So when can you actually stop taking your wheat grass, colloidal minerals, probiotics and evening primrose oil?

Listen very carefully to the answer…

NEVER! Let me repeat that again … *NEVER, NEVER, NEVER!*

The only time you need to stop having these supplements is when they stick you in a box and bury you in the ground (or reduce your corpse to ashes)!

These foods and supplements are **not** like a prescription that you get from your doctor and only take for a few weeks or months. These are something that you take <u>for the rest of your life!</u>

Please don't forget this.

Important Final Note...

If you are currently suffering from a serious "nutritional deficiency" disease or ailment then you may need to supplement with extra nutrients and utilize the benefits of additional therapies.

For this particular form of diagnosis and guidance, I would strongly recommend you read the book *Lets Play Doctor* by Dr Joel Wallach and Dr Ma Lan (available from Amazon).

It describes the symptoms and treatment modalities for over 400 different diseases and conditions using natural medicine and vitamin/mineral therapy.

An absolutely superb book, which I believe should be in every household in the country!

The Forgotten Cure: Natures Natural Antibiotic - Olive Leaf Extract (OLE)

Before we move on to our healthy eating plan (number two of our health and longevity program), I would first like to talk about some of the amazing benefits of the nutritional marvel known as olive leaf extract. Even though this hasn't been included in our supplementation program, I believe it would still be a worthy addition to the program for many people, particularly during the beginning phase.

New research has shown that olive leaf extract can assist tremendously with many of today's common health problems.

Amazingly, many people still haven't heard of OLE, and yet it's been used as a natural antibiotic for thousands of years. Only recently, since the active components in olive leaf extract were isolated, has its popularity resurfaced and some remarkable discoveries been uncovered.

Research by the Upjohn Company (now owned by Pfizer) and published by the *American Society for Microbiology,* found that the active components in olive leaf extract (oleuropein, hydroxytyrosol, elenolic acid and calcium elenolate) were able to inhibit the growth of every virus, fungi, bacteria and protozoa they were tested against (they tested more than thirty microorganisms). [44,45]

This means that olive leaf extract is beneficial for controlling bacterial and viral infections that cannot be controlled through the use of antibiotics; including coronaviruses, cold and flu, encephalitis, Epstein-Barr, herpes, pneumonia, dengue fever, severe diarrhea, many sexually transmitted diseases, and fungal problems such as candida and tinea.

OLE is also able to control the antibiotic-resistant micro organisms that have now been created from the overuse of antibiotics (something many of the "experts" believed could never happen). [44]

Olive leaf extract works on viruses by interfering with critical amino acid production - which is needed for a virus to grow. OLE is able to penetrate infected cells and halt viral replication. [44,45]

With bacteria, olive leaf extract is thought to actually "dissolve" the outer lining of the microbe. It not only helps to contain the spread of any such infection, it also strengthens the immune system dramatically. [44,45]

In Hungary, OLE has produced exceptional results for treating a wide range of infections, so much so that it's now considered an official anti-infectious disease treatment by the government. [44,45]

In 1992, French Biologists found that olive leaf extract was able to either inhibit or kill all of the herpes viruses (genital herpes, cold sores, shingles, etc). More recently, virologist, Dr Harold Renis was able to confirm this finding and discovered that the main active ingredient in olive leaf extract, oleuropein, was what actually killed the virus. [44,45]

Expert biochemist, Arnold Takemoto, had this to say about olive leaf extract... *"it (olive leaf extract) sure has power; particularly against viruses that are more tenacious! It fills a hole that we haven't been able to fill before. It gives us a new and effective tool."* [55]

At the University of Southern California Medical Centre, Dr W.J. Martin, who is head of molecular immunopathology at the centre, found that a high number of patients who suffer from Chronic Fatigue Syndrome have very unusual retroviruses in their bodies.

Other studies on CFS have shown that this condition is closely associated with immune dysfunction. This dysfunction is what allows various microorganisms (parasites) to invade and grow in the body, which in turn causes chronic infection. [44,45]

Because olive leaf extract is able to strengthen the immune system and kill the growth of these microorganisms, its potential for combating Chronic Fatigue Syndrome looks very promising.

Another area that looks promising regarding the use of olive leaf extract is in the treatment of HIV and AIDS. Dr Morton Walker in his book, *Olive Leaf Extract*, has documented cases of patients with HIV and AIDS who were able to alter their HIV antibody status from positive to negative with olive leaf extract. [44,45]

In one case, a HIV patient was able to decrease his viral load from an exceedingly high 160,000 organisms per millilitre of blood down to 30,000 in only a couple of weeks. Over the next eleven weeks, it progressively fell to an astonishing 692! [44,45]

More Powerful Benefits of Olive Leaf Extract...

Olive leaf extract has many additional benefits aside from its antiviral and antibacterial activity.

It's extremely good for the heart and circulation and helping to prevent the oxidation of LDL (bad cholesterol). OLE is also able to relieve heart arrhythmia (irregular heartbeat) and increase blood flow to the heart. [44,45]

Italian researchers found that olive leaf extract reduces hypertension and lowers blood sugar levels and uric acid levels in animals, which indicates a possible treatment for diabetes and heart disease in humans. [44,45]

Australian researchers also found olive leaf extract to be lethal to human prostate cancer and breast cancer cells in laboratory testing. OLE has an antioxidant capacity that is 400% higher than Vitamin C and almost double that of green tea and grape seed extract. [46]

One of the first benefits usually noticed by someone taking olive leaf extract after the first few weeks is a substantial increase in energy. As the microorganism load on the body is decreased, energy levels begin to rise.

The great thing about olive leaf extract is it's safe and non-toxic to the body. The only "side-effect" - if you can call it that – which you may experience for the first few weeks of taking OLE is the die-off effect (Herxheimers reaction once again). This occurrence is simply the death and eradication of harmful parasites and pathogens from the body (which is a good thing).

So, for the first few weeks you may actually feel worse before you start feeling better. Once you get over this hurdle though, you'll begin to feel better, perhaps better than you've felt in a long time.

If there was only one supplement/natural antibiotic that you decided to keep in your medicine cabinet, this would surely be it!

Taking olive leaf extract at the onset of an infection and then continuing until the infection clears will ensure a quick and strong recovery.

If you suffer with any of the ailments already described in this section, including a lack of energy, then I would suggest that you take olive leaf extract at the beginning of the program in conjunction with your wheat grass and other supplements. After 12-14 weeks you can then stop taking your OLE and just keep it in the fridge for emergencies - or instead, take it for a full month every 3-6 months to give your body a regular parasite cleanse (like I do).

#2 - The Healthy Eating Plan: Good Food for Good Health

Now that we're ready to have our all-important foods every day, we need to have a look at a basic eating plan for each day.

When it comes to the consumption of food, keep this thought uppermost in your mind. It's always better to eat five or six small meals a day rather than the traditional three large meals. Because the body can only assimilate and use so much food at a time, any extra just puts more stress on your organs, makes you feel tired, and causes the excess calories to be stored as body fat (yes, small regular meals will help you lose weight).

You'll also notice in this section that I do not give set amounts of how much food you should eat for each meal. The reason for this is there are many different factors that determine how much food one should eat in a day. For example, your body size, whether you're pregnant or breastfeeding, and the most crucial one, your metabolism!

Some people have a fast metabolism and so will need to consume more calories than someone with a slow metabolism.

The type of work you do is another factor. Someone who has a very physical job is going to burn more calories than someone who sits behind a desk all day.

If you exercise regularly then you will likewise burn more calories, and as a result, will need to eat more than someone who's a couch potato.

So what I've done here is given recommendations on what to eat for each meal, but left the amounts up to you.

It's very simple to work out how much you should be eating for each meal though.

Here's a few simple guidelines:

• Only eat until you feel slightly full but satisfied.

• Don't eat until you feel as bloated as a pregnant goldfish!

• Small, light meals throughout the day are the key.

• Remember that each meal should also contribute in some way to the supplying of nutrition to the body. This means nutritionally dead foods are out and nutritionally alive foods are in!

THE MORNING

I'm sure you've heard it said many times that breakfast is the most important meal of the day.

Although I believe that *every* meal is the most important, there is some truth to this statement.

Your body has been fasting for at least eight to ten hours while you've been asleep and it's depleted. It's in desperate need of some good quality food to get it going for the day.

So around twenty minutes after having your wheat grass and other supplements, it's time to eat!

***Foods in for Breakfast*:** Unprocessed cereals, fruit, natural yogurt, kefir milk, chia pudding, eggs.

***Foods out for Breakfast*:** Sausages, bacon, traditional pancakes, hash browns, etc.

There are a number of healthy *and* incredibly tasty foods that can be eaten for breakfast.

Obviously, foods like sausages and traditional pancakes (except keto pancakes) are out (and with good reason) and foods such as cereals, fruit, kefir milk, natural yogurts, and yes, eggs, are in.

These foods are not only packed with real goodness, they're also easily digestible, which means your body won't feel sluggish in the mornings.

When it comes to choosing a breakfast cereal, it's important to choose a natural cereal such as organic raw oats or bran or uncooked muesli rather than a processed cereal like Wheatabix or Cornflakes (raw, unprocessed cereals are far more nutritious than processed ones).

Something as simple as some raw organic oats (non GMO of course) with kefir milk or almond milk, along with a tablespoon of LSA mix or teaspoon of chia seeds or hemp seeds sprinkled on top makes a delicious and nutritious start to the day.

Or what you can do instead is make up your own healthy muesli. Find a herbal/health food store that stocks dried goji berries, pepitas, coconut flakes, chia seeds, hemp seeds, crushed almonds and

Why we Should Avoid all White Flour Products...

Here's yet another example in which man has taken a wholesome natural food and totally messed it up through refining and over-processing.

White flour (used to make breads, etc.) is made from wheat that's been chemically treated and altered - to the point where it's unrecognisable from its original form.

The bran and wheatgerm is first removed, along with all of the valuable nutrients. The remaining flour is mostly "nutrient-dead" starch.

Chemicals such as chlorine, peroxides, and a substance called azodicarbonamide are used to bleach the flour and prevent any fungus growth (which by the way, also destroy the friendly bacteria in our intestines when we consume them). Once flour has been bleached, it essentially becomes a type of sugar.

And if this is not enough, more chemicals including emulsifiers, extenders and improvers are used so the bread has a smoother texture, stays fresher longer and looks more attractive. Finally, when the bread is "as white as toilet paper" it's ready for us to eat! [14]

If you want to enjoy good health then it's imperative that all white flour products be avoided. Wholemeal flour is a natural and far better alternative so try and go with this instead.

When it comes to bread, the best investment you can make is to buy a home bread maker. You can then bake your own bread using wholemeal flour, linseeds, rye, or any of the other healthy grains. Making your own sourdough bread is another healthy option. Just keep in mind that too much bread isn't good for you, so be sure to eat it in moderation.

raisins. Mix 1-2 cups of each in a large container filled with organic oats (this will be your stored amount to keep in the pantry). Half to one cup of this mix for breakfast each morning with some kefir milk or almond milk is mega healthy and tastes yumo!

If on the other hand, you decide to have fruit for breakfast then make sure it's fresh fruit and not tinned fruit. Tinned fruit contains little in the way of nutrients and usually comes with added sugar. Some freshly chopped fruit in a bowl with yogurt and kefir milk on top also makes a delicious and nutritious breakfast. If you cannot find fresh fruit, snap frozen fruit is the next best option.

Finally, if you choose to have eggs then these are best eaten either soft boiled, poached or scrambled. Never fry them.

Mix and Match...

So there are a number of options you can have when deciding what to eat for breakfast.

You could have just one of the foods discussed every morning, or you may choose to have a different one, or maybe a combination of two or three of them. It's totally up to you.

For instance, you might decide to have cereal one morning and then eggs on sourdough toast the next. Or, you might choose to have a combination of cereal and some yogurt for the same meal. Or you might decide to have a little bit of everything. The choice is yours.

What's important is that you have a variety of foods to choose from so you don't become bored with what you're eating. As they say, variety is the spice of life!

Oh, and one last thing.

Please, whatever you do, do not skip breakfast.

So many people miss this important meal and don't realize the consequences until later on in life when their body starts to break down. Even if you only have something small like a piece of fruit, it's certainly better than just having a cup of coffee or nothing at all.

MID-MORNING

Foods in for Mid-Morning Meal: Fruit, yogurt, salad, vegetable juices.

Foods out for Mid-Morning Meal: Biscuits, cakes, chips, soft drinks, etc.

What you decide to eat for this meal will usually depend on what you ate for breakfast.

I would recommend something simple and light like fruit and/or natural yogurt.

If you already had these for breakfast, however, then you might choose to have something different like a small Caesar salad with natural dressing or a tossed salad.

In addition to this, I would recommend having a glass of fresh fruit/vegetable juice (e.g., carrot and celery, carrot and beetroot with ginger, cucumber with apple and celery, banana with apple and kale). There are some excellent websites out there with plenty of simple and easy juicing and/or smoothie recipes. Just search online to find them.

If you're not feeling hungry at this time, then you can just have the vegetable/fruit juice or smoothie on its own if you choose. Remember, raw vegetable juice is high in nutrients and important live enzymes. For this, having a juice extractor or NutriBullet/NutriNinja in the kitchen or workplace is a must. (If you're unable to have the raw vegetable juice at this time, you can always have it at another mealtime).

LUNCH TIME

***Foods in for Lunch*:** Salad, vegetables, rice, pasta, sourdough bread, tofu, eggs, tuna, chicken, salmon.

***Foods out for Lunch*:** Pies, sausage rolls, pasties, hamburgers, chips, fried foods, etc.

Once again, there are a number of options to choose from when deciding what to have for this meal.

For instance, you could have something simple like a tuna/salmon and salad sourdough sandwich, or a chicken and salad sandwich, or even just a plain salad sandwich with sourdough bread.

Or you might prefer a Caesar salad or a tossed salad (with a sprinkle of LSA on top) with black rice, egg, tuna or chicken.

Or what about a falafel salad or tofu and egg salad?

Maybe you'd prefer some steamed black rice or fried rice (not cooked in oil) and vegetables instead.

There are many different combinations and this is where some good healthy eating recipe books come in handy (there are dozens out there to choose from) as they do a wonderful job of making seemingly boring foods highly appetising.

MID-AFTERNOON

***Foods in for Mid-Afternoon Meal*:** Fruit, vegetables, seeds (pumpkin, sunflower, psyllium, chia, etc.), nuts (almonds, walnuts, cashews).

***Foods out for Mid-Afternoon Meal*:** Ice cream, chocolate, lollies, biscuits.

This meal, as with the mid-morning meal, is best kept light and simple.

Something like a piece of fruit, or a small fresh fruit salad, or some raw vegetables (either juiced or whole) along with a few raw seeds or nuts would be ideal.

The beauty about these foods is they continue to help us sustain our energy levels at the time of day when we can sometimes start to feel a bit lethargic.

EVENING MEAL

***Foods in for Evening Meal*:** Vegetables, salad, rice, pasta, meat (lean beef, chicken, fish), legumes (chickpeas, soya beans, lentils), eggs, tofu, sourdough bread, herbs (garlic, ginger, parsley, alfalfa, etc.)

***Foods out for Evening Meal*:** Sausages, chops, salami, fried foods, pies, processed foods, junk food, etc.

What you have chosen to eat throughout the day will no doubt have a bearing on what you decide to have for your evening meal.

Once again, this is where a good healthy eating cookbook becomes essential. These books can help take a lot of the guesswork out of deciding what to prepare and how to prepare your evening meal. You can also find some great recipes and tips online.

So what are some of the foods you could have for dinner? (After you've had your wheat grass/barley grass and other supplements of course.)

What about a chicken and vegetable stir-fry?

Or some grilled fish with steamed vegetables and mashed potato?

Or yummy falafels (my personal favorite) with a vegetable stir-fry and baked potato?

Or what about a lentil meatloaf (don't knock it until you try it!) or delicious black rice risotto?

Maybe you'd prefer home made spaghetti bolognaise or a tuna and pasta salad perhaps?

If you like spicy foods then you might enjoy a hot vegetable and lentil curry or some spicy cauliflower buffalo wings?

I could keep going on about the different food ideas, but I think you get the picture. The bottom line is there are literally *hundreds* of healthy recipes and food combinations to choose from.

As I said, all it takes is a little imagination and a good cookbook or recipe to make your evening meal not only healthy, but also very satisfying.

AFTER DINNER SNACK

If you find yourself feeling a bit peckish a few hours after your evening meal, I would suggest something small and light like some fruit, nuts, chia pudding or natural yogurt (I like it frozen).

Alternatively, as an after dinner treat you might like to have some home-made ice cream (it's easy to make) or churn up some frozen banana, mango or berries using a Yonana (online search it). This terrific appliance makes healthy frozen desserts at home with a minimum of fuss. It's definitely one of our favorite kitchen appliances!

With whatever after dinner snack you decide to have, just remember to keep it small.

Other Important Health Tips...

One substance that no human being can survive even a few days without is of course, water.

Our bodies need water for a variety of functions including the removal and flushing of toxins and chemicals, along with the transporting of vital nutrients. Without enough water, the cells in the body shrink from dehydration and the cell membranes begin to dry out.

It's therefore extremely important that we drink plenty of pure filtered water (at least eight to twelve glasses) every day.

Now, notice I say "filtered" water.

Don't believe for one second that our tap water is clean, and therefore, safe. Tap water is known to contain a cocktail of chemicals, pesticides and additives including sodium fluoride (rat poison), pharmaceuticals such as artificial hormones, antibiotics and mood stabilizers, along with other drugs – this according to a recent Associated Press investigation. [3]

The only way you can make sure the water you're drinking is clean is by first filtering it.

Also, thirst is a very poor indicator of when your body is in need of water. By this time, you're already dehydrated. So make sure you drink plenty of water at regular intervals throughout the day to keep yourself hydrated.

Something else that people pay little attention to but is very important for our health and wellbeing is our breathing.

We don't consciously think about the way in which we breathe, but if we did, most of us would soon realize that we spend most of our waking hours breathing shallow rather than taking in full breaths. Shallow breathing does not supply the body with a full amount of oxygen.

We know that oxygen is vital for the functioning of the human body (we can go days without water, months without food, but only minutes without oxygen), so it makes sense to take in as much oxygen as you can for every breath you take!

Do you know that diseases such as cancer cannot survive in an oxygenated environment? It *can* survive quite nicely in a poorly oxygenated or acidic environment though. This is another reason why calcium, magnesium and boron are so important to the human body as these key minerals neutralize acid – which in turn helps to keep the body oxygenated.

I'm a big believer in moderate exercise (non-strenuous forms) and one of the main benefits of exercising is that it forces you to breathe full, deep breaths.

So begin to make a conscious effort every day to breathe in and out fully and after a while you won't even have to think about it - it will just happen naturally.

In addition to this, I recommend you look up the Wim Hof Breathing Method. This technique has helped me in so many wonderful ways - particularly in becoming more focused, helping me sleep better, and boosting my energy levels. The difference it makes is quite amazing.

The last important health item we need to make sure we're getting enough of is obviously, sleep.

The amount we each need every night varies from person to person, but it should be in the vicinity of seven to nine hours.

If you aren't getting enough sleep then you'll definitely find yourself feeling tired and lethargic during the day and you may even begin to experience health problems as a result (a lack of sleep lowers the body's immune response).

If you've ever been ill, you'll know that rest and sleep are vital for recovery. Sleep is also what helps the body to recover from the work it's had to do during the day.

It's therefore essential that we all make sure we're getting the necessary amount of ZZZ's our bodies need every night.

Finally, we need to look at the one thing we want to make sure we **don't** get enough of... stress.

This horrible condition causes more health problems than most people realize. In fact, it can literally kill you!

When you're under stress, the body releases toxic chemicals into the bloodstream. If you remember back to when I was talking about enzymes (chapter 8), and how we only have a limited supply - and how stress uses up that supply prematurely - you'll appreciate just how crucial it is to keep our stress levels under control.

We must learn to relax!

And what are some ways to do this?

In the next chapter I talk about meditation, which is a fantastic way to relax and lower your stress levels. Exercise is also a great way to relieve stress and let off some steam, so to speak. Taking what I call regular "time out" breaks can help to keep stress levels under control as well.

In Summary...

When working out what to eat for each day, remember that your diet should consist of around 60-70% fruits, vegetables and herbs, 20-30% legumes, whole grains, seeds and nuts, and around 10-20% meat and eggs.

Also remember to only eat small light meals, spaced roughly two and a half to three hours apart, and drink plenty of filtered water regularly throughout the day.

Furthermore, try and buy organically grown produce where possible and avoid all processed foods.

And most importantly, *don't forget to have your supplements everyday!*

#3 - Exercise... Not Just for a Healthy Bod!

Now, here's an activity some people avoid like the plague.

Good old-fashioned exercise!

I don't know why though because it makes you feel so much more vibrant and alive and better about yourself. Exercise not only keeps your body healthy; it keeps your mind healthy as well.

You see, when you exercise your brain releases powerful chemicals called endorphins. These chemicals have a mood stimulating effect, which means you feel happier, think clearer and enjoy a heightened sense of awareness.

Another benefit of regular exercise is the physical aspect. When you're fit and in-shape you feel good about yourself and this positively affects other areas of your life. You also become more relaxed and think more positively, which in turn improves your work and family life.

Certainly, the other major benefit of regular exercise is the health aspect. It's a well-known fact that exercise and remaining active helps you live longer. The heart stays strong, many diseases are prevented and joint mobility is greatly improved through regular daily exercise... as long as you don't overdo it.

I'm constantly amazed at how many people are out there busting their buns everyday, exercising like a mad man (or woman) and sweating like crazy, and actually believing they're keeping themselves healthy.

All they're doing is shortening their lifespan dramatically!

Consider this: when you exercise hard and push yourself to the limit, you put your nervous system under tremendous stress. And when you sweat you don't just sweat out salt and water, you sweat out <u>all</u> of the essential nutrients.

If strenuous exercise was good for you then elite athletes should live the longest, shouldn't they?

Except, there's *never* actually been an elite athlete live to be a hundred years old.

Not one... zippo, zilcho!

More people have actually dropped dead on a basketball court than in a boxing ring. And how many elite athletes have suffered life threatening health problems such as irregular heartbeats or myocarditis and had to retire early?

Believe it or not, strenuous exercise actually kills more people around the world than car accidents. [7,27]

So be sure to think about this interesting piece of trivia before you go out and exercise till you're about to vomit!

Best Forms of Exercise...

What are some of the best forms of non-strenuous exercise then?

I think going for a brisk walk is still the number one choice. Walking is easy to do and doesn't put any strain on the joints like running or jogging does.

I do stress though that it needs to be a "brisk" walk so that the heart rate is increased. You should basically be at a level where you're puffing but could still carry on a conversation if you had to.

Around 40 minutes a day, 4-5 days a week would be sufficient. Naturally you should start off slowly, and as your fitness level increases, gradually increase the amount and pace of your exercise program.

I find that hiking, or even something as simple as taking the dog for a walk down the local park, is not only great exercise, it's very relaxing as well. There's something about being with nature that makes you feel peaceful and tranquil and at ease with life.

I believe it's important that we all have some time to ourselves to just relax and put our minds in neutral for a while. Walking is great for this!

Cycling is another safe form of exercise that you can do. Cycling is low impact as well and because it helps to keep the knee joints lubricated, it can benefit people who suffer with knee problems.

Swimming is also extremely good and great for the joints, particularly the elbow and shoulder joints.

Weight training is yet another form of exercising that's extremely beneficial. Studies have shown that people who suffer with arthritis respond very positively to this type of exercise program. This is due to the fact that weight training helps to slow down bone loss, lubricate the joints, strengthen the surrounding muscles, and reduce the pain and inflammation associated with arthritis.

Regular weight training sessions will also help you lose unwanted body fat and tone and shape your body. And ladies, please don't think that you'll end up "muscly" if you train with weights. I don't know why most women seem to think that if they weight train, they'll end up looking like a steroid enhanced Ms Universe contender!

Training with weights will tone your body... that's all.

The other forms of exercise that have become popular these days are fitness classes such as Pilates, Grit, bootcamp, aqua aerobics and step.

These types of exercise regimes are certainly okay as long as they're low impact and not excessively strenuous. Just remember to always wear good comfortable shoes when doing any type of aerobic fitness session (except aqua-aerobics of course!).

Tips for Losing Weight

While I'm still on the subject of exercising, here's a few extra tips for anyone trying to lose weight...

Understand that if you're trying to shed those unwanted pounds then you don't just need to limit your fat intake (except essential fatty acids as these will help your body burn body fat), you need to limit your intake of high sugar/high starch carbohydrates as well (especially after 3pm).

Many people have the mistaken belief that fat in the diet is what makes you overweight and by cutting out all fats, you'll lose weight. They don't realize that eating too many carbohydrates will make you overweight also! Whatever carbohydrates (particularly sugars and quick burning starches) the body doesn't use or burn off are stored as body fat.

Also, try to eat as many raw foods as possible (especially lots of grapefruit as this fruit contains an enzyme that helps the body burn fat).

Research by Dr Edward Howell showed that cooked foods over-stimulate our glands, particularly the pituitary gland and pancreas, causing an over release of insulin. This causes us to gain weight, whereas raw foods are non-stimulating. This non-stimulation effect results in the maintenance of normal (and healthy) insulin production, and in turn, a normal healthy weight range. [12]

A healthy functioning liver is also important for anyone trying to lose weight as this organ is essential for regulating carbohydrate/sugar metabolism and fat metabolism. The beauty of the wheat grass, colloidal minerals and evening primrose oil is they're all super powerful liver tonics and liver cleansers!

Best Time to Exercise...

As a final note on losing weight, bear in mind that exercising first thing in the morning, before you've had anything to eat (tea or coffee is okay), will bring about the quickest results.

The reason for this is your body has no food left to use for energy (it's been fasting for the last 8 or so hours), so it will burn body fat for energy instead.

Additionally, try not to eat for at least half an hour after exercising as the body will continue to burn body fat at this time.

When it's time to have your shower, have a warm shower to begin with, then for the last 30-60 seconds, switch to cold only. Yes, it's going to be freezing! The benefit of this is cold water helps the body burn fat, as several studies have confirmed.

This is another part of the Wim Hof Method... cold showers every day. It works!

* * *

In Conclusion...

So that concludes *The Ultimate Health and Longevity Program.*

Remember that the three main elements of this program are: supplementation, correct diet, and exercise.

For this program to be successful, you need to utilize all three.

For many of you who already live a fairly healthy lifestyle, this will be easy.

For others who are – how do I say it – "not being so kind to their bodies," this may be a little more difficult.

Just be sure to begin slowly and make some small lifestyle changes every day. And of course – be positive.

You can do it!

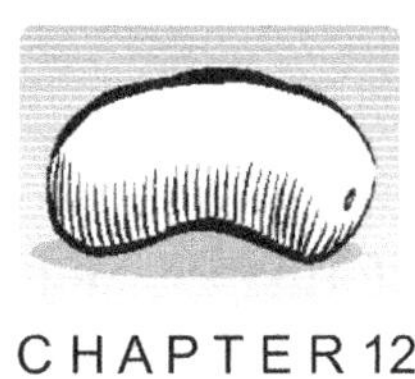

Some Final Thoughts and Ideas...

In this, our final chapter, I would like to share with you some thoughts and ideas that I believe will not only help us on our path to obtaining the fabulous health and longevity benefits we're seeking, but will also help us all to enjoy a wonderful and purposeful life filled with prosperity, abundance and real happiness.

We don't just want to be healthy and live longer. We want to get the most out of life and enjoy all it has to offer as well, don't we?

Well, there are some things that we can do to help us discover this truly incredible and fulfilling side of life. A side of life that we may not believe is even possible for us to live, or may not know exists for us in the first place!

So here are some ideas that we can use to help us on our journey...

1. The Ancient Art of Quieting the Mind

If you were to study all of the wisest and most influential teachers and masters that have existed down through the ages, from the great Buddha to Mahatma Ghandi to the Dali Lama, you would discover that all of them practised some form of daily relaxation or meditation.

These people seem to have instinctively known the value of spending time every day just quieting the mind and listening to the universal voice inside.

When we as human beings do this, we are able to tap into a unique and vast source of endless information and inspiration.

Many of the world's great works of art and inventions and scientific discoveries were conceived by individuals during a state of total relaxation.

One of the all time great inventors, Thomas Edison, is reported to have spent time everyday in a state of total relaxation. Apparently, he would have a pen and note pad next to him and would awaken at various times, write something in his note pad, then lie back down. Many times he couldn't even remember doing this but said that this practice was responsible for many of his inventions.

I also remember reading about a prominent billionaire who said he never makes any important business decisions without first meditating on them.

When we relax the mind, information and inspiration come to us easily and effortlessly. Naturally, it's something that as we continually practice more and more, we get better at.

The other major benefit of daily meditation is not only does it relax the mind, it relaxes the body as well. In fact, one hour of meditation is equal to around three hours of sound sleep.

After you've finished a meditation session, you feel totally at peace and on a "natural high." It really is difficult to describe the sensation you feel. The mind is also much clearer and sharper and you're able to focus and concentrate much more easily.

Now, please understand that meditating does not mean wrapping yourself up like a contortionist and reciting the word "omm" over and over until you're blue in the face. (Although you can certainly do this if you so choose).

Meditation is simply relaxation. Sitting down on a chair, closing your eyes and totally relaxing the body and mind. Having some relaxing music going softly in the background while meditating also helps.

By concentrating on your breathing (breathing in slow full breaths and exhaling slowly and fully), you begin to go down deeper and deeper into a state of wonderful and blissful relaxation.

So begin to make a habit of meditating every day and you'll notice almost immediately just how much more relaxed, calmer and less stressed you are. It really is a marvellous feeling!

If you want to find out more about meditation or yoga or other relaxation techniques, there are many books available that can help you. Or alternatively, you can go to classes that are run by professional and experienced teachers. I also recommend searching "The Teachings of Abraham" by Jerry and Esther Hicks on YouTube. These powerful, guided meditations and videos have had an enormous positive effect on my life – and I know they'll do the same for you.

2. Purpose, Direction and Fulfilment

The great Leonardo da Vinci once said... *"A well spent day brings happy sleep. A well spent life brings happy death."*

How true that is, and this important statement leads me into the next topic I believe is vital to each and every one of us: the importance of finding purpose and direction in our lives.

I find that human beings are really strange creatures. We go through life chasing after the things that don't really matter and neglecting the things that do matter.

How often has someone on "deaths bed" expressed remorse for

not spending enough time with their family, or wasting their life and not really finding out what they were here to do in the first place? (Or what Dr Wayne Dyer refers to as your "heroic mission").

No one ever says, "I wish I had of made more money," or "I wish I had of bought that Porsche I always wanted." We all know that these things are insignificant when you look at the bigger picture.

Life is more than working to accumulate a whole bunch of worthless possessions. It's about making a contribution; to your fellow human beings, and to this wonderful planet on which we live.

You see, I believe that each and every one of us has been put on this planet for a reason – a purpose. And it's up to each of us to discover that purpose.

If you go through life enjoying wonderful health and longevity, but don't make something of your life or find your purpose in life along the way, then I believe you've done yourself a great injustice.

And it doesn't have to be something grand like saving us from nuclear destruction, or ridding the world of starvation. It could be something simple like going down to your local old people's home and helping out, or providing shelter for homeless animals, or helping out your favourite charity organization.

Whatever it is, it's up to you to find it. And it's really not that hard to discover what your purpose is.

Just follow your heart and do what you love!

If you love plants then go open a nursery. If you love kids then become a day care worker. If you love helping people then become a counsellor, or a volunteer for the Salvation Army. If you love birds then go open an aviary. If you love to ride horses then go and start your own horse-riding club. If you love to make people laugh then go and be a stand-up comedian.

It really doesn't matter what you do as long as by doing it you make the world a better place and you enjoy it.

Don't go through life hating your work – waking up Monday wishing it was Friday. Discover your purpose, do what you love, and life will take on a whole new meaning!

Now, I know what you're probably thinking at this point. You would like to do what you love except you have commitments, right?

How can you just give up what you're doing when you've got bills to pay and food to put on the table?

Well, what if you just start out doing it in your spare time and see what develops? The exciting thing about life is that you just never know where it might take you!

Oh, and here's something else to keep in mind when finding your purpose.

It never, ever involves money or taking advantage of another person. If you do something for these reasons then you're doing it for the wrong reasons.

If you're able to make loads of money out of doing what you love then great. If you don't then that's great also because you're still on purpose and enjoying what you're doing.

Let's face it, we all have a choice. We can either sit back and watch life happen or we can go out and make life happen.

I recommend the latter.

Remember too that with whatever work or career you choose to do, make sure you don't neglect your family.

Instead of chasing that extra sale or doing that extra bit of paperwork or working those extra hours, go home!

Spend some time with your kids. Play ball with them. Go for a ride on your bike with them. Take your spouse out on a date. Go and visit your parents. Spend time with the people you love.

No matter how long we live, there are still only so many tomorrows.

3. The Life-Changing Power of Books

I remember going to a seminar many years ago and hearing the great Charlie "Tremendous" Jones speak. It was a fantastic experience and certainly worth every ounce of money that I paid.

The one thing I never forgot about that seminar was a powerful statement he made at the very beginning. He said: *"You'll be the same person in five years as you are today except for two things: the people you meet and the books you read."*

Boy is that true!

All of us have had people who have come into our lives and affected us, either positively or negatively. Some have helped us and some have hurt us.

We have always been warned to "be careful of the company we keep" or that "you become like the people you associate with."

There's no doubt that the people you meet and associate with throughout your life can make all the difference to the type of person you become and where you go in life.

Of course, the other thing that will make all the difference is "the books you read."

And this doesn't mean books like Mills & Boon or Stephen King. It means personal development books and books that help to expand your knowledge and help you gain wisdom and understanding.

The beauty of these books is you can learn from people who are either a professional in their field or have already experienced what they're writing about.

For example, if you wanted to know how to become financially independent then you could read a book on that subject by someone who's already achieved that.

If you wanted to become more self confident then you could read a book on how to become a more confident person.

If you wanted to be able to understand your partner better then you could read a book on personalities or relationships by someone who deals in that area.

If you wanted to be able to deal with people better then you could read a book on how to do that.

The list is endless, and the wonderful thing is there's virtually a book out there to help you with any and every life situation that you could encounter.

There have been many influential people through the ages who have said that reading books changed their lives. Steve Jobs, Bill Gates, Warren Buffet, Elon Musk, Oprah Winfrey and Barack Obama are just a few of the more recent.

I particularly enjoy reading biographies and stories of people who've done great things or have overcome great obstacles. You can learn so much from these people. And what's good about reading their stories is you can gain some of their wisdom and insight from just a few weeks (or days) reading.

You don't have to go through what they've experienced to gain what they've gained.

That's powerful knowledge!

They say that the average person reads one book a year, so if you read ten books a year then you'll be ten times smarter and more knowledgeable than the average person, right?

Look, there are basically two ways in which you can learn and gain knowledge. You can either do it by trial and error, which is tough. Or you can learn from other people's experiences and expertise.

It makes a whole lot more sense to me if you can learn (primarily) from other people's experiences and know-how. It can save a heck of a lot of time and unnecessary heartache.

Naturally, you're still going to make mistakes and have ups and downs. That's a part of life. However, through the reading of books, you can help stack the odds of success greatly in your favor!

And what about the cost of buying all these books you may ask?

Think of it as an investment.

I would have to say that what I've learnt and the person I've become over the years from reading positive-inspired books has been worth a thousand times more to me than any money I've had to spend on buying them.

If you can't afford to buy books then an alternative would be to join your local library. Most local libraries stock an excellent range of inspiring and personal development books.

I sincerely hope that you will take the time to invest in your own mind and your own future and *read! read! read!* It will be one of the best and most rewarding decisions you ever made.

Where Will You be in 5 Years Time?

Think about this: the next five years are going to happen, whether you like it or not. You're going to be somewhere in five years time, aren't you?

If you look at where you were five years ago, that will give you a pretty good indication of where you'll be and the person you'll be in another five years.

If you don't like the thought of that then you need to change some things, and it all begins with what you feed your mind. This book has primarily been about what to feed your body, but understand that what you feed your mind is just as important.

So begin today to read positive and inspiring books and in five years time you'll be truly amazed at the person you've become and grateful for the life that you live!

Where to Begin...

Probably the biggest challenge you'll have with reading books is knowing where to start and finding the right ones. There are just so many out there to choose from.

What I will do then is give you a list at the end of this section of some of the books that have had the greatest impact on my life, and the lives of many people I know, and you can start with these if you like.

Keep in mind though that because we're all at different stages in our lives, we will relate to some books more than others. You may read a book for the first time and get little out of it, yet you go back and read it again six or twelve months later and it all makes perfect sense.

I think that the more we read, the more our level of awareness expands.

I also find that many of the books we need to read and the ones that will have the greatest impact on our lives are drawn to us exactly when we need them.

For instance, I remember when I first read the book, _Reaching for Heaven_.

The timing for that was perfect.

Just a few weeks before I bought the book a close friend of mine had been tragically killed in a plane crash. Up to that point in my life I had taken many things for granted, and like most people, was caught up in my own little world.

After the accident though I began to seriously question a lot of things… about life, and about death. There were a lot of questions that were unanswered, and a lot of things that just didn't make sense to me.

Suffice it to say that everything I needed to know at that point in my life was contained in that book. I know that if I had of read it six or twelve months earlier it wouldn't have had the same impact as it did.

What can I say? The timing was perfect.

There are also books out there that will change *your* life for the better. You just have to be open and receptive to them and know that they will come to you when the time is right. This book itself may have even come into your life at the exact time that you needed it.

I don't believe anything happens by chance.

My Top 10...

Okay then, here's a list of some of the books and audiobooks that I feel will be of tremendous benefit to you.

Like I said though, you'll probably relate to some books better than others, so if you read a book or listen to an audiobook and find that it just didn't do it for you then simply put it away for the time being and try reading or listening to it again at a later date.

By the same token, I believe that even if you only get one piece of wisdom from a book then it has still been well worth it!

1. ***Being Happy, Making Friends*** **and** ***Follow Your Heart*** **by Andrew Mathews**

These three books really are fantastic and great starter books. Everyone can relate to what Andrew writes about and they're also very easy to read (with lots of amusing cartoons throughout each book). I remember reading a story about former professional golfer Nick Faldo and how he attributed his victory in the 1992 US Open to the reading of the book *Being Happy*. I would easily consider these three books to be amongst the top ten best personal development books ever produced.

2. *You Are What You Think* by Doug Hooper

This is also a fantastic book on overcoming obstacles and making the most of your life. There are many stories of hope and triumph from people Doug helped over the years, including convicts and ex-convicts that many believed were a lost cause and could not be helped or rehabilitated.

3. *Your Erroneous Zones* by Dr Wayne W. Dyer

The all time classic and record-breaking bestseller about you and your personality. This is perhaps the best book that has ever been written on how to be and achieve all that you've ever wanted. Some of the subjects covered include: how to stop worrying about what other people think, getting rid of the "fear of failure" mentality, and how to develop assertiveness and self confidence. Definitely one to keep in your book collection!

4. *How to Win Friends and Influence People* by Dale Carnegie

Another all-time classic on how to understand and deal with people in every area of life. This book is a very easy read with lots of interesting stories. What I find incredible is that even though it was written over eighty years ago, the information it contains is still very relevant today!

5. *Men Are From Mars, Women Are From Venus* by Dr John Gray

Most people have already heard of this book, but not many have actually read it. It's a great book for anyone who's involved in a relationship as it gives invaluable advice and understanding on how to get along with your partner better. I know that if all couples read this, divorce rates would easily be halved!

6. *You'll See It When You Believe It* and *Your Sacred Self* by Dr Wayne W. Dyer

These are two extraordinary and life-changing books on discovering the inner self. I guarantee that once you read them, you'll never look at life and the universe in the same way again. Be prepared to experience a wonderful sense of inner peace and clarity in your life that you never thought possible!

7. *The Secret, The Power* and *The Magic* by Rhonda Byrne

Featured on the Oprah Winfrey show and also New York Times bestsellers, these phenomenal books have changed the lives of millions around the world. They not only explain very simply how you can have anything and everything you want in life; they also explain how it all comes about and how the magnificent "magical" process works. Three incredibly powerful books!

8. Becoming Supernatural by Dr Joe Dispenza

Even Tony Robbins says that this is one of the greatest books of all time. So much power and wisdom is contained in this book. What I love about Dr Joe Dispenza is he's a doctor and a scientist, so he doesn't just explain how you can become "supernatural," he proves his workings and findings through the powerful brain measuring equipment that's used in his seminars. Another New York Times bestseller which definitely deserves a special place on your bookshelf.

9. The Power of Now by Eckhart Tolle

If I had to pick the ONE book that truly changed my life, my thinking, and the way I view my inner and outer world (and myself), this would surely be it. This is one of Oprah Winfrey's all time favorite books; so much so that she became, and continues to be, a powerful advocate for its teachings and had much to do with it selling well over a million copies and being translated into 30 languages. All I can say is whatever you do, DO NOT pass up reading this book!

10. *Conversations With God* (Books One, Two and Three) by Neale Donald Walsch

I've definitely saved the most controversial ones for last. Amazingly, these books have probably created more uproar (particularly in the religious field) than any other book written in the last one thousand years!

Neale Donald Walsch had a direct "conversation with God" that lasted on and off for six years and produced three books, which are all New York Times bestsellers and have sold over seven million copies worldwide, along with being translated into 32 languages. Every question that humans have ever wanted to ask "God" since the beginning of time is asked and answered in intricate detail, from "is there extra terrestrial life" to "what about sex" to "global warming and the environment" to "is there a hell and did Hitler go there."

What I love about these books is all of the information contained in them makes perfect sense. Be warned though, sometimes the truth can be a tough pill to swallow. But as the great book says … "know the truth and the truth shall set you free!"

Other Books Worth Reading...

Louise Hay was a beautiful soul and acclaimed author of many outstanding books on self healing and loving of the self. Her most famous "You Can Heal Your Life" has sold an astonishing 50 million copies (and counting). Be sure to devour her books and audio's as much as you can!

Neville Goddard was one of the true pioneers of modern day thinking and one of the originators of the law of attraction. I would strongly encourage you to read all of his books or listen to his amazing audiobooks, particularly "Feeling is the Secret."

Jerry and Esther Hicks (The Teachings of Abraham) also have some terrific books and audio titles that I highly recommend, especially "Ask and it is Given."

Books that inspire and give us hope are always fantastic reading as well.

Biographies on people who have done great things or have had to overcome great obstacles in order to achieve in life can help us to do the same. When you read about these people you realize that they are human just like you.

You start to think that if they can achieve something worthwhile or overcome adversity and still live a purposeful life then maybe you can too. They begin to give you something that is very important... belief!

Other books that are also fantastic reading are the *Chicken Soup For The Soul* series. These books contain inspirational and touching stories of everyday people who have managed to overcome obstacles and setbacks in life and yet still triumph and achieve greatness.

They're the type of books that once you start reading, you find it very hard to put them down.

Needless to say, there are many other books out there that will benefit you on your life journey. I've only suggested a few of them. It's important that you spend lots of time in bookstores and online sites such as Amazon, Booktopia and Barnes & Noble checking out the various book and audio titles they have available.

Finding Time

I know the hardest part for many of us is being able to find the time to read them all. I personally find that setting aside some reading time everyday enables me to read the books I want.

For instance, reading for twenty or thirty minutes before going to sleep or twenty or thirty minutes upon awakening might be the perfect time.

Or instead of watching TV every night or sitting on your phone or iPad, read for half an hour or so during that time instead (you will benefit more from a good book than you will from some of the garbage that's on TV and social media anyway!).

If you travel, particularly to and from work, instead of listening to the same old music or radio station, why not listen to a good quality audiobook instead?

Whatever time you do choose to read though, just be sure to make a habit of doing it ***every day***.

YouTube, Dailymotion and Vimeo...

I would also encourage you to spend lots of time on YouTube and/or Dailymotion and Vimeo and watch some of the highly informative video's and seminars by Dr Joe Dispenza, The Teachings of Abraham (Jerry and Esther Hicks), Louise Hay,

Neville Goddard, Eckhart Tolle and Dr Wayne Dyer, to name a few (you can also find these people or groups associated with them on Facebook and Instagram).

What I love about these platforms is there are SO many handy video's - and they're all free (you just have to put up with the annoying ads). If you're not a big reader, watching video's is a great alternative.

In Summary...

These three ideas: daily meditation, finding and doing what you love, and the reading of positive books, I guarantee will make all the difference to your life.

In fact, show me any successful person and I'll show you someone who practices these ideas on a daily basis.

It takes effort to succeed in life, that is true, but it also takes effort to fail as well. If you do these three things every day, you will succeed – of that you can be certain!

Life is a Series of Choices, and our Lives are the Result of the Choices we Make

Now I know not everyone would agree with that statement, but it's true.

No matter what happens to us in life, we all have a choice on how we deal with our circumstances and which road we decide to take when presented with either an opportunity or a challenge.

What I find really amazing is how one person will learn and benefit from a situation, while another, presented with the same situation, will give up and/or take the negative path.

There's a story about two brothers that's a perfect example of this…

They both grew up with a very violent father who would constantly beat them and their mother – sometimes until they were almost unconscious.

This man had no respect for anyone or anything and eventually ended up in jail for armed robbery.

Thirty years later a magazine decided to do an article on the two brothers and separately interviewed both of them to find out what they were doing and how they had turned out after such a traumatic childhood.

The first brother had unfortunately turned out exactly like his father and was currently serving time in jail for armed robbery.

The second brother, however, had a successful career and was happily married with three children. He was, in fact, one of the most kind and loving people you could ever meet.

When the interviewer asked the first brother why he turned out the way he did he answered: "Well, look at my childhood, what do you expect!"

What's really interesting though is that when the interviewer asked the second brother the same question, he replied: "Well, if you look at my childhood you'll see why."

Two people, same circumstance. One chose to learn and benefit from the situation while the other chose to continue on the same negative path as his father.

I believe you are now faced with a similar choice.

You can either choose to take everything that I've talked about in this book and use it to your benefit, or you can choose to ignore it and continue on your present path.

Or you might choose to use only some of the ideas presented in this book and not bother with the rest.

I know some of the ideas may seem a little silly, or even ridiculous, but that's only because they're unfamiliar to you and not everybody you know uses them.

At least give them a go!

What have you got to lose?

I know that if you do, you'll look back on this time of your life in years to come and say: "That was the turning point. That was the time when my life really began to change for the better."

Robert Frost, in his wonderful book *The Road Less Travelled*, sums up what I'm trying to say very well:

Two roads diverged in a wood,
and I took the one less travelled
by, and that has made all the
difference.

You can make a difference. Not just to your own health and your own life, but to the health and lives of many other people as well.

When you begin to feel healthy and look healthy, and have a positive outlook on life, people want to know what you're doing differently.

They can't help but want to know.

And of course, when they do, hand them this book!

Give them the same opportunity to benefit as you have had.

It really is great if we're able to benefit from something; it's even better if we can help other people to benefit from it as well. And when we do this, we not only feel good, we are also living the abundance principle, which means that when you give something to someone without any thought of return, you receive back tenfold!

…You can begin today on the exciting path to abundant health, prosperity and real happiness.

You can also become a positive role model for many other people, including your family, just by doing one simple thing – making the choice to do so.

And you can choose to make that choice right now – if you choose to!!!

In Conclusion...

Wow, I can't believe we've already come to the end of the book.

There has certainly been a lot of information covered and it's important that you now go back over the main chapters and re-read them.

"Repetition is the mother of all learners" and this book is not one that you read once and then put away like you would a novel. It's a book that you continue to read and refer to over and over and use as your "health guide."

I remember a prominent businessman telling me that you haven't read a book unless you've read it at least three times. This is good advice.

In closing, I would like to briefly answer the number one question that I get asked by people I meet... "Why did you take the time to write this book?"

The simplest answer I have been able to give is: "To help save lives."

This book was written out of a sincere desire to help people.

Like I said in the introduction, I do not claim to have all the answers – not by a long shot. But I do know one thing. What I've discussed in this book works, and works extremely well!

Writing, researching and putting it together has also been a monumental task for me, taking over ten years, on and off, and what little spare time I had to complete. There were many times along the way when things just didn't seem to be going right and I felt like giving it away (I accidentally erased my manuscript at one point and had to start again).

What kept driving me though was my dream…

My dream of seeing a society of people who are no longer sick and tired and filled with disease and despair, but instead, are enjoying the vitality and radiant health and longevity that we as human beings are all entitled to.

A far off dream it may seem to some, but when you realize that people are now more health conscious than they've ever been before and are now seeking natural alternatives for their health problems more than ever before, this dream doesn't seem so far off.

William James once said: *"Nothing is more powerful than an idea whose time has come."*

Well, the time for this idea has certainly come.

It's time for us to make "healthiness" our way of life instead of allowing the body to slowly wither and degenerate through misuse and neglect.

I believe you now have the information you need to do exactly that – to make healthiness *your* way of life.

But remember, information is useless unless it's put into practice.

You must make the necessary effort yourself. No one else can do that for you.

I sincerely hope that you do take the information given and use it. If you do, then my job has been worthwhile and your money has been well spent.

From this day on... *your* health and *your* life are in *your* hands!

I wish you all the best.

Review and Rating...

Dear valued reader. I sincerely hope you gained something of value from this book. If you did then you will have richly rewarded me more than you could ever know.

If this book has managed to help you then I would be most grateful if you took a quick moment to leave a review and star rating on Amazon. This would also help to "get the word out" to others.

You can leave your feedback by either scanning the QR code below or visiting your Amazon orders page.

Thank you very much… and have a wonderful day!

Exclusive Bonuses

Included in the purchase of this book are four additional ebooks… *How to Take off the Pounds and the Years, Nutritional Secrets to More Youthful Skin, How to Boost Brain Capacity Naturally* and *The Truth About a More Exciting Sex Life.*

To gain access to these, log on to www.lifesavinghealth.org/bonus-material

Bibliography and Footnotes

1 Wallach, Joel, Dr, *Dead Doctors Don't Lie*, informational cassette tape, 1995.

2 Bragg, Paul C and Patricia, *Apple Cider Vinegar*, Health Science, p.8 & 93.

3 Bullivant, Vaughan, *The Natural Way to Better Health and Longer Life*, pp.2-9, 18-19, 29-44.

4 Sustainable Agriculture and Food Enterprises Pty Ltd, informational video.

5 Aussie With Heart Conquers North Magnetic Pole, Australian Heart Foundation brochure.

6 Trudeau, Kevin, *Natural Cures "They" Don't Want You to Know About*, Alliance Publishing Group, 2004, p.10.

7 Wallach, Joel, Dr, *Hell's Kitchen*, informational compact disc, 2004.

8 Posner, Howard, Dr, *A Live Doctor Telling The Truth*, informational cassette tape.

9 Wallach, Joel, Dr, *Dead Doctors Don't Lie*, Wellness Publications LLC, 1999, p.30 & pp.143-160, 60-66, 386-387.

10 Wallach, Joel, Dr, *Have You Heard?*, informational compact disc, 2005.

11 Udall, Kate, *Amino Acids-The Building Blocks of Life*, Woodland Publishing, 1997, pp.5-9, 11-19.

12 Swope, Mary, Dr, Green *Leaves of Barley*, Swope Enterprises, 1987, p.24, Quoting David.A. Darbro, MD, pp.42-49, 52-56, 112-124, 127-134, 145-155.

13 Anton, Bill, B.S.C., *Colloidal Minerals-Natures Best Kept Secret*, Woodland Heath Series, pp.5-17, 19-22, 23-39.

14 L 'Abbe, Bert, Dr, and Connery, Chuck, Ph.D, *Forbidden Secrets*, informational cassette tape, LP Recordings P/L.

15 Pietsch, Russell, (DDA,B Th), article from June/July edition of *Natural Life Review* magazine, 2004, p.28.

16 S.A.F.E. Pty Ltd, *Our Friends the Lactobacilli Family* (exert taken from *Fighting Fatigue* by Dr Ian Brighthope), informational brochure.

17 Lifelong Vitality newsletter, June 2004.

18 Wallach, Joel, Dr, *What's Up Doc 2*, informational cassette tape, 2004, Total Nutrition.

19 Wallach, Joel, Dr, *Live Doctors Do Lie*, informational cassette tape, 2001.

20 Schrauzer, Gerhard, Dr, *Selenium-The Inside Story*, informational cassette tape, LP Recordings P/L.

21 Strand, Raymond, Dr, *The Medical Evidence That Demands a Verdict*, LP Recordings P/L.

22 Natural Facts Pty Ltd, *Zinc The Superstar of Minerals*, informational brochure.

23 Readers Digest, *Foods That Harm Foods That Heal*, 1997, pp.40-41, 150-151, 237-241, 360-367.

24 *Sustainable Agriculture and Food Enterprises PTY LTD*, informational brochure.

25 Downs, David, *Free Radicals and Antioxidants*, Willowbridge Massage Clinic, 1996, pp.1-4, 14-15.

26 Wallach, Joel, Dr, *Medical Milking Machine*, informational cassette tape, 2002.

27 Wallach, Joel Dr, *Medical Dogmas and Lies*, informational cassette tape, 2000.

28 Seibold, Ronald, M.S., *Cereal Grass-Natures Greatest Health Gift*, Keats Publishing Inc, 1991, pp.18-32, 36-48, 55-75, 79-83.

29 Lee, Deborah, *Essential Fatty Acids*, Woodland Publishing Inc, 1997, pp.5-11, 16-23, 26-29.

30 Bradstreet, Karen, *Evening Primrose Oil*, Woodland Publishing Inc, 1997, pp.6-18, 23-27.

31 O'Hara, Peter, B.A., Dip. Hom, *The Perfect Food For Health*, informational article from S.A.F.E. Pty Ltd.

32 McDonnell, Ziema, Dr, Health and education article, S.A.F.E. Pty Ltd.

33 Australian Council For Responsible Nutrition Inc, *The Supplement-Antioxidants and Aging Effects on Memory* section.

34 S.A.F.E. Pty Ltd., promotional newsletter, Nov, 1995.

35 O'Hara, Peter, *Herbal Fibre Formula*, health article, S.A.F.E. Pty Ltd., promotional literature.

36 O'Hara, Peter, S.A.F.E. Pty Ltd., promotional literature.

37 O'Hara, Peter, B.A. (Hons), Dip Hom, *Green Barley*, article which appeared in Silver Cord magazine, May, 1997.

38 O'Hara, Peter, *The Green Green Grass of Home*, S.A.F.E. Pty Ltd., promotional literature.

39 Tenney, Deanne, *Acidophilus*, Woodland Publishing, 1996, pp.5-7, 12-19

40 Tenney, Louise, *Colon Health*, Woodland Publishing, 1998, pp.10-15, 21-24.

41 World Environmental Conference and the Multiple Sclerosis Foundation F.D.A. issuing for collusion with Monsanto, article written by Nancy Markle (1120197).

42 Stoddard, Mary Nash, *Aspartame-The Deadly Deception*, informational cassette recording.

43 Treffers, Sue, *Food Additives-A Pocket Sized Reference to Their Use, Origin and Effects*, Hartrade Pty Ltd., 1999, pp.7-86.

44 O'Hara, Peter, B. A. (Hons), Dip Hom, *Olive Leaf Extract-Natures Antibiotic*, S.A.F.E. Pty Ltd., promotional literature.

45 *Natural Life Review* magazine, June, 1999, article entitled *Olive Leaf Extract a Natural Alternative to Antibiotics.*

46 Complimentary Healthcare Council, *Retailers News* brochure, produced by John Pye, CHC retail division general manager and Kate Hannon, CHC communications and media manager.

47 NCBI, PubMed, Randomised trial of coconut oil, olive oil or butter on blood lipids and other cardiovascular risk factors in healthy men and women, published March6, 2018.

48 cocoveda.net, Study Shows Heart Disease Absent in Coconut Eating Population

49 Simon, Michele, *Is the Dietitians Association of Australia in the Pocket of Big Food?*, EatDrinkPolitics.

50 American Lung Association website article, *The Impact of E-Cigarettes on the Lung.*

51 mercola.com

52 Morgan, Graeme, Ward, Robyn, Barton, Michael, The contribution of cytotoxic chemotherapy to 5-year survival in adult malignancies, PubMed, National Library of Medicine.

53 Steven E Coutre 1, Megan Othus, Bayard Powell, Cheryl L Willman, Wendy Stock, Elisabeth Paietta, Denise Levitan, Meir Wetzler, Eyal C Attar, Jessica K Altman, Steven D Gore, Tracy Maher, Kenneth J Kopecky, Martin S Tallman, Richard A Larson, Frederick R Appelbaum, Arsenic trioxide during consolidation for patients with previously untreated low/intermediate risk acute promyelocytic leukaemia may eliminate the need for maintenance therapy, PubMed, National Library of Medicine.

54 NCBI, PubMed, Treatment of erectile dysfunction with pycnogenol and L-arginine, Published May/June 2003.

55 Fourwinds Nutrition Inc USA, Olive Leaf Extract Concentrate health article,

Made in the USA
Monee, IL
08 July 2026

56564653R00154